Geriatric Medicine: an
evidence-based approach

Geriatric Medicine: an evidence-based approach

Edited by

Frank Lally

Christine Roffe

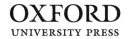

OXFORD
UNIVERSITY PRESS

OXFORD
UNIVERSITY PRESS

Great Clarendon Street, Oxford, OX2 6DP,
United Kingdom

Oxford University Press is a department of the University of Oxford.
It furthers the University's objective of excellence in research, scholarship,
and education by publishing worldwide. Oxford is a registered trade mark of
Oxford University Press in the UK and in certain other countries

First Edition published in 2014

Impression: 2

Published in the United States of America by Oxford University Press
198 Madison Avenue, New York, NY 10016, United States of America

British Library Cataloguing in Publication Data
Data available

Library of Congress Control Number: 2014941934

ISBN 978–0–19–968964–4

Printed in Great Britain by
Clays Ltd, St Ives plc

Dedication—Prof. Peter Crome

Peter Crome has worked in the National Health Service, academic institutions, and professional bodies since 1970. He has led the development of clinical and academic geriatric medicine in local, regional, national, and international arenas. As head of Keele Medical School, chair of the Geriatrics Committee of the Royal College of Physicians, president of the Section of Geriatrics and Gerontology of the Royal Society of Medicine, secretary general of the Clinical Section of the International Association of Geriatrics and Gerontology, and president of the British Geriatrics Society, he has given strategic direction to the development of geriatric medicine nationally and internationally.

Peter has inspired a generation of geriatricians by promoting clinical excellence, bringing a research ethos into every aspect of clinical practice, and encouraging others to develop a wider vision and positive approach. His influence has been pervasive. Through the Master's degree in Geriatric Medicine he founded at Keele University, academic seminars and conferences, and mentoring of students nationally and internationally, he has shaped a generation of geriatricians. As president of the British Geriatrics Society, he has been instrumental in changing the clinical specialty of elderly care into the academic discipline of geriatric medicine.

The chapters in this book are inspired by Peter's interests and are written by experts in the field in celebration of his work. They reflect Peter's wide influence within the specialty of geriatric medicine and the impact that he has had upon it. His research includes publications on pharmacokinetics in older people, stroke, dementia, involvement of older people in clinical trials, addiction, mental health, pain, and frailty, with seminal papers and book chapters in all of these fields. His interests have not just been theoretical. He has carried his studies through into improvements in clinical practice, undergraduate and postgraduate education, and policy implementation. Peter is not only an incisive thinker; he also has the ability of making things happen in complex circumstances and difficult situations.

No one who knows Peter can fail to appreciate his optimism, realism, humour, unfailing humanity, and his broad smile. However, most of all, he is a devoted doctor, a trusted colleague, and an intuitive mentor, always eager to be supportive and inclusive.

With all of Peter's admirers it would have been possible to fill this book several times over. As it is, the chapters collected here will stand as a token of the affection and esteem in which he is held by all of his friends and colleagues.

Preface

While it is fashionable to lament the perceived future adverse impacts of increasing longevity on society, health care provision, and social services, such doom may be misplaced, as increased longevity is a consequence of better health, and life years gained may be productive and contented. While the recent increase in retirement age can be seen as a purely economic expedient, it also reflects the realities of better health in older people. Nevertheless, towards the end of life, at whatever age this occurs, frailty, memory loss, pain, and multimorbidity are likely to remain problems encountered in years to come as they are now. Evidence on the effectiveness of preventative and therapeutic interventions is increasing rapidly, and approaches to treatment of the older person are changing apace. With more age-related problems becoming treatable or preventable, simply caring for the elderly is no longer an option.

More than in any other specialty, the way the service is delivered and how support is provided in the community are important determinants of health and quality of life in this population, and new models of care are being developed.

This book will give the reader a grounding in current thinking in geriatric medicine, highlight the research which has led to changes in management strategies, point to key sources of up-to-date information on the topic, and probe into questions that still remain to be answered.

The contributors to the book are leading UK specialists in their subject areas. Chapters are written in a concise and economical style that conveys the latest evidence-based practice in the treatment of older people along with expert interpretation of the research literature from a specialist's perspective. Learning points and illustrations are provided where relevant, as well as up-to-date references for further material, including useful websites.

The book is an easily accessible reference tool for a broad cross section of health professionals who manage older patients in both primary and secondary care, such as geriatricians, general practitioners, nurses, therapists, and clinical researchers, as well as specialists in pain, stroke, dementia, and palliative care services. The topics and issues raised will be of particular interest to professionals involved in the development of health and community services for older people.

What emerges is the complexity of the care of older people requiring collaboration between multiple agencies along with integration of services underpinned by robust channels of communication. Good quality clinical trials are increasingly providing us with effective interventions to treat many of the conditions of old age. Such advances need to be used to influence care provision at the level of policymakers. In addition, legal and physical infrastructures associated with the provision of care of older people, such as access to services and treatments, require updating and enhanced inclusivity. This book is both a guide to best practice and a manifesto for further improvements of evidence-based medicine for the older person.

Frank Lally and Christine Roffe

Acknowledgements

We would like to gratefully acknowledge the tireless support of Professor Ilana Crome in the preparation of this book and the help of Dr David Roffe in the editing process. We are also thankful to Mrs Kathryn McCarron for ensuring the smooth running of the conference where the germ of this book took root. The production of a book is always a difficult process, but Eloise Moir-Ford at OUP has made this as painless a process as possible and we are most grateful for her patience and understanding.

Contents

Contributors

Dr David Anderson
Consultant Old Age Psychiatrist &
Associate Medical Director,
Mersey Care NHS Trust,
Liverpool Clinical Business Unit,
Mossley Hill Hospital,
Park Avenue,
Liverpool,
Merseyside, UK

Dr Richard Atkinson
Consultant Psychiatrist
for the Elderly,
Lancashire Care NHS Foundation
Trust,
Charnley Fold,
Cottage Lane,
Bamber Bridge,
Lancashire, UK

Dr Roger Beech
Reader in Health Services Research,
Institute for Primary Care
and Health Sciences,
Keele University,
Staffordshire, UK

Prof. Alistair Burns
Institute of Brain, Behaviour
and Mental Health,
The University of Manchester,
Manchester, UK

Prof. Ilana Crome
Hon. Consultant Psychiatrist South
Staffordshire and Shropshire
Healthcare NHS Foundation Trust,
Emeritus Professor Keele University,
Hon. Professor Queen Mary
University of London,
London, UK

Prof. Peter Crome
Research Department of Primary
Care and Population Health,
University College London,
London, UK

Prof. Joe Harbison
Associate Professor of Medical
Gerontology,
Trinity College Dublin,
Dublin, Republic of Ireland

Prof. Stephen Jackson
Department of Clinical
Gerontology,
King's Health Partners Academic
Health Sciences Centre,
Denmark Hill,
London, UK

Dr David Jolley
Honorary Reader,
Personal Social Services Research Unit,
The University of Manchester,
Dover Street,
Manchester, UK

Ms Zena Jones
Senior Manager,
NIHR Clinical Research
Network: Stroke,
Biomedicine West Wing,
International Centre for Life
Times Square,
Newcastle upon Tyne, UK

Prof. Lalit Kalra
Department of Neurosciences,
Academic Neurosciences Centre,
King's College London,
London, UK

Prof. Paul V. Knight
Director of Medical Education
(Associate Medical Director),
Consultant Physician Medicine
for the Elderly,
Royal Infirmary,
Glasgow, UK

Dr Frank Lally
Institute for Science & Technology
in Medicine,
Keele University,
Guy Hilton Research Centre,
Stoke On Trent,
Staffordshire, UK

Prof. Finbarr C Martin
Ageing and Health,
Guys and St Thomas' NHS
Foundation Trust & King's
College London,
St Thomas' Hospital,
Westminster Bridge Road,
London, UK

Prof. Gary H. Mills
General Intensive Care Unit,
Northern General Hospital,
Sheffield, Yorkshire, UK

Sean Page
Consultant Nurse for Dementia
& Senior Lecturer in Dementia
Care Nursing,
Betsi Cadwaladr University Health
Board & Bangor University,
Memory Service,
Wepre House,
Wepre Drive,
Connaghs Quay,
Flintshire, UK

Prof. Chris Phillipson
School of Social Sciences,
Humanities Building,
Bridgeford St,
Manchester, UK

Prof. Christine Roffe
Stroke Research,
North Staffordshire Combined
Healthcare Trust and
Institute for Science & Technology in
Medicine,
Keele University,
Stoke On Trent,
Staffordshire, UK

Prof. Pat Schofield
University of Greenwich,
Centre for Positive Ageing,
School of Health & Social Care,
Avery Hill Campus,
Grey Building,
Avery Hill Rd,
Eltham, UK

Dr Adrian Wagg
Professor of Healthy Ageing,
University of Alberta,
Edmonton,
Alberta,
Canada

Dr Kate Wilde
North Staffs Combined Healthcare
NHS Trust,
Holly Lodge,
Hartshill,
Stoke-On-Trent, UK

Chapter 1

From gut feeling to evidence base: drivers and barriers to the development of health care for older people

Paul V. Knight

Key points

- Major advances in medicine, policy, and services for older people have been made over the past 50 years.
- The numbers of older people in the UK and elsewhere are increasing and will continue to do so.
- This increase has concomitant sociological, medical, and economic challenges that need to be met because they affect the provision of services at all levels.
- These challenges are occurring at a time when resources are becoming scarcer and budgets shrinking.
- Governments are faced with orchestrating infrastructure and policy in this demanding and complex scenario.
- Managers are attempting to do more with less.
- Clinicians and other medical professionals are trying to base treatments on sound evidence-based strategies.
- There is recognition of the need to include older people and the general public in these processes.
- Research may provide us with information that can help resolve these problems.

1 **The emergence of geriatric medicine**

Prior to the NHS, illness and disability of older adults of average or low wealth was largely met by local authority provision. Only acute illness preceded by reasonable good health would have reached the 'proper hospitals' in the voluntary and charitable sectors, including the teaching hospitals. With generally poor housing stock, and little more than family and other informal care to fall back on in the community, institutionalization was a much more common outcome than it is now. The National Health Service Act 1946 was a defining event for older people's care as it brought these large and poorly staffed institutions into a health care oriented universal service. The specialty of geriatric medicine was made necessary by this political act, though it needed early clinical pioneers to give it life.

Meanwhile the National Assistance Act 1948 empowered local authorities to provide accommodation for older people whose frailty, old age, or poverty rendered unable to manage at home. This arbitrary distinction of health and social care was set down in law, and remains a challenge to the provision of a flexible yet holistic approach.

2 **Older people's medicine into the mainstream**

The initial focus of geriatric medicine was people with ongoing disability, mostly in long-stay NHS hospitals inherited from local councils. The buildings often previously served as workhouses. The changes from the 1950s to the 1980s can be summarized as follows:

+ Application of conventional medicine to this previously underserved population of patients rendered many able to recover sufficiently to leave hospital.

+ Early but quite basic developments in rehabilitation and devices reduced disability.

+ Organization of geographical areas under health boards (with various names) brought some order to the distribution of resources and the gradual spread of geriatricians to most areas.

+ Closure of worn-out buildings and the rationalization of dispersed services into larger district general hospitals brought geriatric medical beds into the mainstream, with better access to facilities and staff, notably junior doctors.

+ Facility to admit older people directly, rather than from waiting lists or by transfer from other hospital departments (usually less than satisfactory recovery), gave geriatricians a role in their acute medical care.

- This, along with expansion of social care provision, brought about markedly better outcomes and reduced hospital lengths of stay.

- Closure of NHS long-stay hospitals, plus changes to statutory regulations enabling older people to access various forms of supplementary income, resulted in major expansion of the private and voluntary care home sector. This coincided with a general loss of NHS long-stay beds, particularly in England.

- This privatization had the consequence of transferring medical responsibility for thousands of hitherto 'hospital patients' into primary and community care, with little transfer of the commitment or skills necessary for their care. Thus the focus of geriatric medicine became acute hospital services, with dwindling capacity for day-hospital activity such as elective multidisciplinary assessment.

- The increasing public costs of funding care home places and domiciliary social support associated with inadequate assessment of disabled older people led to the NHS and Community Care Act 1990. This created a framework for better health and social care collaboration.

- Geriatricians' presence on the acute hospital site and better access for older people to higher-tech medicine resulted in many of them developing subspecialty skills and roles (e.g. in stroke, cardiovascular conditions, endoscopy, and orthogeriatric rehabilitation).[1]

3 Demographics

When Marjory Warren published the first of her much-quoted articles in the *BMJ* in 1943 (1), she annotated no references to support her conclusions but drew on her personal observations of the many patients who had alighted in the wards of the West Middlesex County Hospital. One of the main drivers to support her assertion that a modus operandi of care was needed was the fact that the absolute numbers of elderly people in the population was rising and would continue to do so.

The numbers of people over the age of 65 years has continued to increase in the UK and elsewhere. The trend is set to continue according to many national surveys (Box 1.1). This increase in the older population carries with it sociological, medical, and economic burdens that are likely to affect the provision of services at all levels. These challenges are occurring at a time when resources are

---

[1] The author gratefully acknowledges the contribution of historical background information (sections 1 and 2) by Prof. Finbarr Martin.

becoming scarcer and budgets shrinking. Due to the complexity of these challenges, governments alone are unlikely to be able to deal with them. Instead there will likely be a need for collaboration between multiple agencies with integration of services nationally and across different disciplines at multiple levels.

Box 1.1 Ageing statistics

- 'The UK has now reached a point where there are more people over State Pension age than children. By 2020, the Office for National Statistics (ONS) predicts that people over 50 will comprise almost a third (32%) of the workforce and almost half (47%) the adult population'.

Text extract reproduced from Gov.UK (2) under the Open Government License v2.0.

- 'The number of older Americans increased by 6.3 million or 18% since 2000, compared to an increase of 9.4% for the under-65 population. However, the number of Americans aged 45–64—who will reach 65 over the next two decades—increased by 33% during this period'.

Text extract reproduced from Administration on Ageing USA (3).

- The European population over 65 years was 17.5% in 2011 and is projected to be 29.5% by 2060. 'The share of those aged 80 years or above in the EU-27's population is projected to almost triple between 2011 and 2060'.

Text extract reproduced from Eurostat (4) © European Union, 1995–2013.

---

4 Integrated services

Governments and commentators have recognized the fact of an increasing population but have been perplexed as how to best deal with the increased longevity of our Westernized populations. Longevity is seen as a problem rather than a triumph. Lately, the language has been somewhat hysterical and a suggestion has been raised in some quarters that older people are being specifically targeted (5). A survey of health professionals across Europe showed that many, particularly in the UK, felt that ageing was a threat to the viability of individual health systems (6). Initially, geriatricians sought practical solutions to improve the care of older people but lacked the impetus or resources to conduct specific controlled trials; descriptions of successful services were published instead (7). This has led to a diversity of service and much debate about what seems best in different settings. Unlike an organ specialty such as cardiology, geriatric medicine depends not only on the skill and training of its physicians, but the availability of other team members and the relationship the service may have with social care professionals often employed and funded by different organizations. Take a cardiologist from Glasgow to Geneva and the coronary care unit and basis of service setup will be essentially very similar; but take a geriatrician from Manchester to Milan and the same will not be the case.

Physicians have realized that our systems for dealing with multimorbid older patients need a new paradigm (8). Not only that, but if these changes do not come about then hospital care, in particular, will fail (9). Geriatricians have endeavoured over the years to publish trial evidence that proves a particular system of working best benefits older people. They have coined the term *comprehensive geriatric assessment* (CGA) (10–12) to describe what happens, although, as CGA seems to be a black-box assessment, exactly how it acts is still open to debate. The benefits have been variously described until recently, when systematic reviews showed significant and sustained benefits for older hospital inpatients in a variety of acute and restorative settings when they were treated by a dedicated multidisciplinary team in a dedicated area. Benefits included reduction in mortality, reduction in nursing-home admissions, and improved function (10–12). Such evidence is being used to persuade policymakers and health service commissioners to purchase the best care for older hospitalized patients so that, provided certain processes are followed, it can be the same no matter what the geographical location.

5 Frailty and geriatric syndromes

Most organ specialists have the ability to look at treatments specifically designed towards a particular organ outcome; for instance, reduced cardiovascular events in those with triple coronary vessel disease. In geriatric medicine the metric of definition has been harder to grasp until the more recent descriptions of *frailty*, with proponents oscillating between phenotypic and index methods of identification (13). (See also Chapter 7.) In any event, it is clear to most geriatricians that frailty is our basic science and a unifying population description for those who would benefit most from service trials and from specific preventative interventions. Frailty also describes one of the main differences between geriatric medicine and organ specialties, as frailty is the non-specific presentation of disease which has a final common pathway of symptom complexes. Frailty is often described collectively as geriatric syndromes. This leads the unwary into the trap of being unable to distinguish disease modification from the normal ageing process (14).

Bernard Isaacs coined the expression the *geriatric giants* or the four Is: impairment of intellect (cerebral dysfunction), incontinence, immobility, and instability (falls). The term *giant* reflects frequency and enormous burden to sufferers (15). The geriatric giants do not quite translate into the entirety of geriatric syndromes although there is considerable overlap.

6 Legislative frameworks

Although geriatricians espouse treating the whole person within a multidisciplinary construct this still requires the use of specific treatments for organ-specific illnesses. These treatments are often engineered through trials that specifically exclude older people (Chapter 16) and thus lead to the wrong targets for treatments in that specific population (16). This has led to collaborations between geriatricians and organ specialists creating a more realistic view of what treatments can do and how they should be deployed in a frail population; for example, cholesterol-lowering agents (17). However, the exclusion from clinical trials of 'unvarnished free-range older people' remains an obstacle to the use of new pharmaceutical agents. Currently there seems little appetite in Europe to recognize this issue in regulatory agencies.

7 Access to facilities and treatment

Older people are known to have lower treatment rates for most forms of cancer. Geriatricians have used CGA as standard practice for some time. CGA improves outcomes for frail older people and it has now been used with some success in oncology. Improved outcomes have made oncologists more willing to give older, particularly frail older people, access to treatments. Access to treatments in mental health and addictions is, similarly to oncology, poor.

There is a need to be aware of the non-specific presentation of geriatric syndromes and how this affects treatment outcomes. Although outside geriatric medicine the use of CGA is mainly used in oncology, there seems no reason why this approach could not be employed in many other treatment settings such as addiction and mental health, where access to services and outcomes can be equally as poor (18).

8 The utilization of the CGA approach to non-elders

The ethos of geriatricians has developed over time to ensure that the team they lead performs a holistic assessment, considering not only disease entities but also the function of the person and the environment in which they live. Some organ specialists are also now aware that this approach can work for younger patients who have complex needs. Thus the culture of geriatric medicine is simply good medicine (19).

9 **Future directions**

For the future then it is important that geriatricians follow Don Berwick's exhortation that we have the right patient, in the right place, at the right time. To this we need to add that we need age-attuned services and interventions proven to be effective in this demographic group.

10 **Conclusion**

The numbers of people over the age of 65 years has been rising for several decades in the UK and elsewhere and continues to do so. This trend has attendant sociological, medical, and economic burdens that present multifaceted challenges for care providers and governments. The complexity of these challenges will require collaboration between multiple agencies, with integration of services underpinned by robust channels of communication.

The situation is no less complex at the level of health care delivery and physicians have realized that a new paradigm is required. Advances in service delivery need to be made. It has been suggested that without such advances, our medical systems, particularly hospital care, may fail.

Good quality clinical trials are increasingly providing us with effective interventions to treat many of the conditions of old age. Even though many of these interventions are cheap and simple to initiate, they may bring functional benefits for patients as well as reductions in mortality and nursing-home admissions. Such advances need to be used to influence care provision at the level of policymakers.

Legal and physical infrastructures associated with the provision of care of older people also require updating and incorporating into any new models of care. This is particularly so in access to services and treatments, the inclusion of older people in clinical trials, and the involvement of patients, carers, and the public in planning those trials and other services.

We are still endeavouring to make progress in the battle with the 'old' geriatric giants such as incontinence and dementia as well as trying to understand the complexities of the potential 'new' giants such as frailty. However, if we are to continue to be successful and move forward, we need a system that is 'joined up' and future-proof in terms of the services' long-term needs.

Websites relevant to this chapter

National service framework: older people—sets out the government's quality standards for health and social care services for older people.

<https://www.gov.uk/government/publications/quality-standards-for-care-services-for-older-people>

The British Geriatrics Society. History of geriatric medicine in the UK. <http://www.bgs.org.uk/index.php/geriatricmedicinearchive/204-geriatricshistory>

Key guidelines, policy documents, and reviews

The British Geriatrics Society. Comprehensive assessment of the frail older patient. <http://www.bgs.org.uk/index.php?option=com_content&view=article&id=195>

Improving opportunities for older people. <https://www.gov.uk/government/policies/improving-opportunities-for-older-people>

References

1 **Warren MW**. Care of chronic sick. A case for treating chronic sick in blocks in a general hospital. BMJ. 1943;**ii**:822–3.

2 **Department for Work & Pensions**. Improving opportunities for older people. 8 Aug 2013. https://www.gov.uk/government/policies/improving-opportunities-for-older-people

3 **Administration on Aging**. A profile of older Americans: 2012. http://aoa.gov/AoARoot/Aging_Statistics/Profile/2012/3.aspx

4 **European Commission Eurostat**. Population structure and ageing. Oct 2012. http://epp.eurostat.ec.europa.eu/statistics_explained/index.php/Population_structure_and_ageing

5 **McKee M, Stuckler D**. Older people in the UK: under attack from all directions. Age Ageing. 2013;**42**(1): 11–3.

6 **A new vision for old age: rethinking health policy for Europe's ageing society**. © The Economist Intelligence Unit Limited; 2012.

7 **Evans JG**. Geriatrics. Clin Med. 2011, **11**(2): 166–72.

8 **Tinetti ME, Fried T**. The end of the disease era. Am J Med. 2004;**116**:179–85.

9 **Hospitals on the edge**. Report of the Royal College of Physicians. 2012. http://www.rcplondon.ac.uk/sites/default/files/documents/hospitals-on-the-edge-report.pdf

10 **Baztán JJ, Suárez-García FM, López-Arrieta J, Rodríguez-Mañas L, Rodríguez-Artalejo F**. Effectiveness of acute geriatric units on functional decline, living at home, and case fatality among older patients admitted to hospital for acute medical disorders: meta-analysis. BMJ. 2009;**338**:b50 doi:10.1136/bmj.b50

11 **Bachmann S, Finger C, Huss A, Egger M, Stuck AE, Clough-Gorr KM**. Inpatient rehabilitation specifically designed for geriatric patients: systematic review and meta-analysis of randomised controlled trials. BMJ. 2010;**340**:c1718.

12 **Ellis G, Whitehead MA, Robinson D, O'Neill D, Langhorne P**. Comprehensive geriatric assessment for older adults admitted to hospital: meta-analysis of randomised controlled trials. BMJ. 2011 Oct 27;**343**:d6553. doi: 10.1136/bmj.d6553

13 **Strandberg TE, Pitkälä KH, Tilvis RS**. Frailty in older people. Eur Geriat Med. 2011 Dec;2(6):344–55.

14 **Kane RL, Shamliyan T, Talley K, Pacala J**. The association between geriatric syndromes and survival. J Am Geriatr Soc. 2012 May;60(5):896–904.

15 **Isaacs B, Livingstone M, Neville Y**. Survival of the unfittest: a study of geriatric patients in Glasgow. Glasgow: Routledge; 1972.

16 **McLaren LA, Quinn TJ, McKay GA**. Diabetes control in older people. BMJ. 2013;346:f2625

17 **Shepherd J, Blauw GJ, Murphy MB, et al**. Pravastatin in elderly individuals at risk of vascular disease (PROSPER): a randomised controlled trial. Lancet. 2002 Nov 23;360(9346):1623–30.

18 **Maas HA, Janssen-Heijnen ML, Olde Rikkert MG, Machteld Wymenga AN**. Comprehensive geriatric assessment and its clinical impact in oncology. Eur J Cancer. 2007 Oct;43(15):2161–9.

19 **Stroke Unit Trialists Collaboration**. Collaborative systematic review of the randomised trials of organised inpatient (stroke unit) care after stroke. BMJ. 1997;314. doi: http://dx.doi.org/10.1136/bmj.314.7088.1151

Chapter 2

Re-thinking care in later life: the social and the clinical

Chris Phillipson

Key points

- Geriatric medicine developed strong links with social perspectives on ageing during its initial phase of development.
- Geriatric medicine and social gerontology developed along separate paths from the 1970s with the emergence of competing paradigms about the ageing process.
- Fiscal austerity, changes to the welfare state, and the increase of age-related conditions such as dementia create possibilities for collaboration between geriatric medicine and social gerontology.
- Areas for joint work between the disciplines include
  - supporting the development of age-friendly communities
  - rebuilding community services
  - challenging health inequalities.

1 Introduction

The nature and type of care provided to older people has re-emerged as a key topic of concern for government, professionals, and older people alike. In the UK, this has been stimulated by debates around the pace of demographic change, the crisis in standards of residential and hospital care, and the rebalancing of support from public to private care provision. A report from the House of Lords, *Ready for Ageing* (1), concluded that while the UK population was ageing rapidly, 'both Government and society were woefully underprepared'. The report expressed the view that 'longer lives can be a great benefit, but there has been a collective failure to address the implications and without urgent action this great boon could turn into a series of miserable crises' (1). The report set this within the context of major demographic and health changes, including 51% more people aged 65 and over in England in 2030 compared to 2010; over 50% more people with three or more long-term conditions in England by 2018 compared to 2008; and over 80% more people over 65 with dementia (moderate or severe cognitive impairment) in England and Wales by 2030 compared to 2010 (2).

Such developments raise major issues both for the organization of services and for the relationship between the different disciplines concerned with the care of older people. The aim of this chapter is to explore the relationship between two of these: geriatric medicine on the one side, and social gerontology on the other. The argument to be explored is that fostering a closer relationship between them will be essential for developing new approaches to supporting older people within the community and for improving well-being in older age.

To develop this theme, the chapter will examine:

- First, the way in which geriatric medicine emerged, noting its links with research on the social context of ageing.

- Second, the subsequent loosening of this connection will be explored and the reasons assessed.

- Third, the emergence of factors making the case for linking geriatric medicine with social gerontology will be reviewed.

- Finally, the paper will conclude with a number of illustrations of a socially informed care of older people drawing together the various disciplines represented in geriatrics and gerontology.

2 **Geriatrics as 'social medicine'**

The development of geriatric medicine (taking England and Scotland as examples) was forged in a social context which itself had a direct impact on practice and clinical interventions (Box 2.1). The modern history of the discipline has been documented in accounts from the late John Brocklehurst (3) and Barton and Mulley (4, 5). An important connecting theme in the evolution of geriatrics—at least from the 1930s—was the battle of the early pioneers against the 'warehousing' and neglect of older people. Thompson's (6) research in the 1940s, summarized in articles entitled 'Problems of Ageing and Chronic Sickness', published in successive issues of the *British Medical Journal*, illustrated this to powerful effect in an analysis of hospitals in the city of Birmingham. Thompson (6) noted that the words 'medical treatment' could only be used in a narrow sense relating to the 'therapeutic use of rest and drugs, because in the infirmaries no other form of treatment was generally possible'. Similar observations had been made in West Middlesex by Warren who had earlier pioneered the concept of rehabilitation applied to the care of older people.

Box 2.1 The development of geriatric medicine

+ challenging the 'warehousing' of older people
+ the social dimension of geriatric care
+ population change as a social and health issue
+ the community context of ageing and unreported illness.

However, the emergence of geriatric medicine also took place in a context of growing awareness of ageing as a 'social' as well as 'health' issue. This was reflected in research sponsored by the Nuffield Foundation (7) as well as in reports concerning the implications for pensions and related issues of the changes associated with ageing populations (e.g. Phillips Committee (8)). This awareness of the social context of ageing was influential in shaping many of the approaches taken by geriatric medicine in its early phase of development. Indeed, it might be argued that geriatrics, over the period from the late 1940s to the 1960s, drew strongly upon what might be termed sociological observations in developing approaches to the care of older people. This was especially the case in respect of those geriatricians who helped transform the profession in this period.

The previous point can be illustrated through examples from the work of Sheldon, Isaacs, Ferguson Anderson and Williamson and his colleagues. Sheldon's (9) *Social Medicine of Old Age* was based upon 447 home interviews in Wolverhampton (conducted by Sheldon himself), where the health of older people was placed within the context of the families and neighbourhoods in which they lived. Sheldon drew a conclusion from his interviews still highly relevant today: 'To regard old people in their homes as a series of individual existences is to miss the whole point of their mode of life in the community. The family is clearly the unit in the majority of instances, and where such ties are absent they tend to be replaced by friendships formed earlier in life' (9).

Isaacs and his colleagues in their study *Survival of the Unfittest*, based upon fieldwork conducted in the 1960s (10), explored reasons for the admission of older people to a geriatric unit in Glasgow, highlighting social issues—such as the strain on what came to be termed 'informal carers' and inadequate care in the community—as major factors. Anticipating debates in the 1990s around 'informal care', the researchers (10) concluded: 'No one could work with the relatives of the geriatric patients of Glasgow, as we did, without developing a profound admiration for their devotion and self-sacrifice. . . . No one could retain for a moment the absurd, oft-refuted, but still prevalent belief that people don't care what happens to old folk. But still one can ask whether the Health

Service ... should have to depend so much on its unsung heroes and heroines, the middle-aged and elderly housewives'.

The idea of geriatrics as embedded in a community context was further developed through the 'preventive' approach in geriatrics. Examples of such approaches are the drop-in health centre for older people developed by Anderson and Cowan (11) in Rutherglen in Scotland in the early 1950s and the 'case-finding' model of Williamson and his colleagues (12). The latter approach demonstrates what Williamson et al. described as the 'iceberg' of unreported illness and the need to seek out disease in apparently healthy older people—an observation subsequently confirmed in longitudinal studies of ageing (e.g. 13).

This development of a community approach ran parallel with early sociological investigations into ageing populations, notably those by Townsend (14, 15) in studies of family life and residential care. In *The Last Refuge,* Townsend (15) identified social factors precipitating admission to a residential home similar to those subsequently reported by Isaacs et al. (10): for example, 'financial insecurity, social isolation and the absence of subsidiary or secondary sources of help on the part of those living with or near a relative' (15). And sociological research in the 1950s and 1960s on the impact of loneliness (e.g. 14, 16) was also influential in raising concerns about the implications for medical practice of changing family structures (e.g. the rise of single-person households).

3 **Geriatrics and social gerontology: divergent paths**

The strands so far identified suggest the possibility of a geriatric medicine which might have developed strong links with emerging research on social aspects of ageing. Yet the period from the 1970s saw geriatrics and social gerontology take divergent paths as each attempted to gain professional and academic respectability (Box 2.2). Geriatric medicine underwent significant expansion in the UK (all four countries combined): from just four consultant geriatricians in 1947 to 335 in the late 1970s to approximately 1,100 by 2010. However, this was in the context of a continuing need to 'defend' geriatrics given negative views within the medical profession, these surfacing at regular intervals in the period from the 1950s onwards (4, 17, 18). This was reinforced through the steady growth of the welfare state and the treatment of ageing as a form of what Townsend (19) referred to as 'structured dependency' arising though the impact of poverty and 'passive forms of community care'. These elements pushed the emphasis in geriatric medicine towards a more exclusive biomedical approach at odds with emerging sociological or social science perspectives on ageing.

> ## Box 2.2 The evolution of geriatric medicine and gerontology
>
> - the growth of geriatric medicine and social gerontology
> - the development of contrasting paradigms of ageing
> - the impact of the welfare state and the 'structured dependence' of older people
> - insights from perspectives on the ageing body.

At the same time, social gerontology began—from the 1970s—its own period of expansion where it sought to carve out a distinctive space around which issues relating to ageing could be researched and discussed (20, 21). Townsend was a pioneer but there was a significant gap before his research in the 1950s and 1960s was built upon. Research into social aspects of ageing (covering the humanities and social sciences) expanded considerably during the 1970s and 1980s, with contributions from a range of disciplines including geography, history, sociology, and psychology. The theoretical models applied by social scientists to ageing in this period also marked a distinctive break with previous approaches, notably by viewing ageing as socially rather than biologically constructed, this being linked with a significant critique of the limitations of biomedical perspectives on ageing (e.g. 20, 22).

However, social gerontology also developed a range of insights highly relevant to the work of geriatricians. For example, research on the body by researchers such as Twigg (23) and Gilleard and Higgs (24) highlighted, among other things, the extent to which many of the long-term illnesses experienced by older people (including disabling conditions such as arthritis) can lead to a progressive loss of confidence in the body. This may serve to undermine relationships in old age, especially those with family and friends. This research also emphasized the damage caused by making bodies invisible in the environments in which care takes place—a point highlighted in many of the reports of abuse of older people in hospital and residential settings (21). The possibility of a more effective link between social science and geriatric medicine is a theme explored in the final section of this chapter.

4 Gerontology and geriatrics: consensus and cooperation

Although, as suggested in this chapter, geriatric medicine and social gerontology have progressed along rather separate paths, developments in the twenty-first century now provide considerable opportunities for collaboration and joint projects (Box 2.3). The forces encouraging collaboration include:

First, the impact of changes to the NHS (with the Health and Social Care Act 2012) and the drive to reduce public-sector provision of care services (25). Such developments are especially significant for geriatric medicine as a discipline and profession, given that its growth and development in the case of the UK was closely associated with the foundation and subsequent growth of the NHS (5). But it is important for social gerontology as well given that so much of the research effort has been around the evaluation of the range of services associated with the welfare state (21).

Second, the need to confront views which present ageing populations as causing a major economic burden and crisis for European economies. International studies such as the Survey of Health and Retirement in Europe (SHARE) make the point that spending on the old does not 'crowd out' spending on the young (26). Moreover, societies where older people are an increasingly important part of the social structure appear to retain a high degree of generational cohesion (27).

Third, the impact of many of the conditions associated with ageing populations— dementia is a notable example—where collaboration across disciplines will be essential for effective care, and for challenging discrimination in access to treatment and support.

Box 2.3 Factors influencing links between geriatric medicine and social gerontology

- ◆ fiscal austerity affecting welfare states and the shrinking of the public sector
- ◆ perceptions of ageing populations as a demographic burden
- ◆ impact of age-related conditions (e.g. dementia).

5 Linking geriatrics and gerontology: areas for development

What are the possible areas for linking gerontology with geriatrics, working from the factors outlined above? The first argument is for a social medicine of ageing which acknowledges both changes in the life course and the impact of inequality on the lives of older people. Geriatric medicine was founded at a time when 'old age' occupied a relatively short and clearly defined period in the life course. Both aspects have been transformed in the twenty-first century, with a range of transitions affecting people from mid-life onwards and with life expectancy at 65 currently extending to approximately 20 years for women and 17 years for men. These developments suggest new possibilities for research, treatment, and care of older people, stretching across the full range of preventive, acute, and long-term conditions. However, this activity will be conducted across a much broader range of lifestyles than was the case when geriatrics and gerontology first emerged, and in the context of positive aspirations about achieving a long and fulfilling later life. The developments described lay the basis for a new approach to understanding ageing, one in which it will be essential to combine insights from across the full range of disciplines covering geriatric medicine and social gerontology. Carstensen and Fried (28) express the context for this in the following way:

> Population ageing presents a *cultural* problem. The dramatic increase in the numbers of people who are making it into their 80s, 90s and beyond is generating a profound mismatch between the cultural norms which guide us through life and the length of our lives. Humans are creatures of culture. We look to culture to tell us when to get an education, marry, start families, work and retire. Because life expectancy has increased so rapidly, we are still immersed in cultures half as long as the ones we are living.

Incorporating the implications of this point in clinical practice will, however, require practical projects where geriatricians and social gerontologists work together on community- and hospital-based projects. This can be illustrated with four examples:

♦ supporting the development of age-friendly communities (AFCs)
♦ rebuilding community services
♦ challenging health inequalities
♦ uncovering the meaning of later life.

The first area concerns the interaction between health and community location, and the need to build what the World Health Organization (WHO) has termed 'age-friendly environments' (29), i.e. those which encourage 'opportunities for health, participation and security in order to enhance the quality of life as people age' (29). Developing AFCs has become a significant dimension in debates in social policy with various factors stimulating discussion around this topic. Such factors include the impact of demographic change across the global North and South; awareness of the impact of urban change on older people, notably in areas experiencing social and economic deprivation (30); and debates about good or optimal places to age, as reflected in policies to support lifetime homes and lifetime neighbourhoods (31). As highlighted in the EU Summit on Active and Healthy Ageing held in Dublin in spring 2013 (32),

> Where we live, our physical, social and cultural environment, greatly impacts upon how we live and age. The significance of 'place' in all our lives cannot be overestimated. The built environment and neighbourhood networks impact on the quality of all our lives and can make the difference between independence and dependence for all people, but especially for those growing older. Place is inseparable from our sense of identity and this is true for people of all ages, including older people.

The implication of this argument is that we need to bring together the debate about building AFCs with a focus on the need to extend the range and extent of community-based services. An important conclusion from surveys such as the English and Irish longitudinal studies on ageing (e.g. 13) is that the most important effects of ageing are likely to be on increased demands for community-based services. Here, there is compelling evidence that personal, informal sources of care remain vital in providing care for those with disabilities of various kinds. The qualification though is that community-based support operates across a broader range of relationships than is often recognized with, in the words of Pahl (33), 'friends increasingly behaving like kin and kin behaving like friends'. One confirmation of this come from data from the Irish Longitudinal Study of Ageing (TILDA), which found that one-fifth of older people receive some form of help from neighbours and friends. Against this, from a sociological perspective, greater recognition is required of the increasingly fragile nature of community support—especially where localities are themselves under economic and social pressures. One argument, therefore, is for developing what might be called a 'community-based gerontology' which draws upon the age-friendly framework but which looks at how we can achieve greater integration of community services with local social networks, and indeed greater use by older people themselves of the full range of services available.

A community-based approach might also draw upon the work of Marmot and his colleagues (34) who have highlighted the importance of social determinants for addressing disparities in health outcomes for people in varying 'social positions' across the life span. The researchers found that both life expectancy and disability-free life expectancies were considerably lower for people living in neighbourhoods with high levels of deprivation. Examples in the UK included the contrast in life expectancies for men aged 65 and over in the London boroughs of Kensington and Chelsea and Westminster: 22.7 years and 21.2 years, respectively, compared with 13.9 years in Glasgow City and 15.5 years in Manchester and Liverpool. From 2004–2006 to 2008–2010, across all areas in the UK, life expectancy at 65 increased by an average of 1.0 years for men and 0.9 years for women, but with the gaps between areas increasing over this time (35). In response to such differences, Marmot argues for actions over the lifespan, from early childhood health and good education through to work opportunities and healthy communities, together with health promotion and support from health and social services.

The central message in the work of Marmot and his colleagues is that actions to improve people's life chances, particularly if taken early in life, can improve health outcomes and address inequalities. Research on healthy ageing is demonstrating that action taken on behalf of people at older ages can also combat social disadvantage, facilitate social well-being, and enable continuing contributions to the communities in which people live (36). While socio-economic disadvantage is largely determined earlier in life, the foundations of adequate income along with affordable and secure housing can still be achieved in old age. The socio-economic resources that can enable people to buy into housing and neighbourhoods and pay for transport reflect lifelong inequalities (37). Social class will be a major influence on healthy life expectancy; i.e. the number of years a person can expect to live free of disability. A life course approach recognizes that it is never too late (or too early) to respond constructively to divergent life chances even as more people live into their 80s and beyond.

Finally, a major challenge which will require joint work across all the disciplines concerns thinking about the meaning of old age and especially late old age in complex global societies. There is much criticism of the professional context within which care and treatment is carried out. Much of this reflects issues about the proper resourcing for care—whether in the community or in hospitals. But it may also reflect the struggle of professionals to accommodate to the distinctive character of longevity. Although late modern society demonstrates that life can be improved in many important ways, human life in general and human ageing in particular pose more questions than science can answer. Here, we need to develop meaningful ways of managing situations in life that in many respects *cannot* be controlled. Conditions such as dementia pose a particular challenge in this regard. By the time someone aged 90 years or more dies, the risk of being demented is approximately 60% (38). But late modern cultures of ageing often have difficulty acknowledging and *dignifying* this reality. Following this, Peter Whitehouse (39) suggests that in the case of conditions such as Alzheimer's the way forward is to rely less on the promise of genetically based therapies, more on the importance of re-thinking the social narrative with which Alzheimer's is associated. He argues:

> Just as all diseases (even so-called 'psychological' ones) have a biology, so, too, is every disease socially constructed. We debate and discuss and then agree (or not) on the labels we use. Saying that something is socially constructed is not to say that the condition is not real or that suffering cannot result from the phenomenology. Rather, the concept of social construction offers the hope that reframing how we think about [in this example] aging-associated cognitive challenges can lead to improvements in the

quality of life of those suffering today and those who will suffer in the future. ... Do we remove the hope when we are more realistic about the likelihood of cure and more effective therapies? No, we create a true hope that puts the responsibility of addressing brain aging in the hands of ourselves and our communities rather than in the domain of pseudoscientific and scientistic prophecy (39).

6 **Conclusion**

Whitehouse's insight offers a significant set of opportunities for geriatricians and gerontologists to work together to build—with older people themselves—a different type of ageing than was characteristic of much of the twentieth century. Then, later life was all too often experienced as a form of dependency underpinned both by negative views about the prospects for change and discrimination within care settings. Such characteristics are still present in the twenty-first century, and may indeed continue given pressures facing health and social care. But new paradigms need to be developed, built around collaborative work between geriatricians and gerontologists. O'Neill (40) makes the point that in a world that is rapidly ageing and short of the expertise of geriatricians and gerontologists, a 'clear definition of roles and close co-ordination between geriatric medicine is required to convince government and international agencies that the sciences of ageing offer the best possible hope to maximize the longevity dividend of collective ageing'. The next decade should see a range of multi- and interdisciplinary projects that should lay the basis of a distinctive and ambitious gerontology and social medicine for later life. Participation across the disciplines and with older people themselves will be a crucial task in the years ahead.

Websites relevant to this chapter

<http://britishgerontology.org/>

<http://www.ilcuk.org.uk/index.php/home>

<http://www.jp-demographic.eu/>

<http://www.futurage.group.shef.ac.uk/home.html>

<http://www.micra.manchester.ac.uk/>

<http://www.who.int/ageing/age_friendly_cities_network/en/>

Key guidelines, policy documents, and reviews

Beard, J., Biggs, S., Bloom, D., Fried, L., Hogan, P., Kalache, A. and Olshansky, J. Global population ageing: peril or promise. PGDA Working Paper No. 8. World Economic Forum: Global Agenda Council on Aging. (2012)

Medical Research Council. A strategy for collaborative ageing research in the UK: developed under the auspices of the Lifelong Health and Wellbeing Programme London: MRC (2009).

Phillipson, C. Ageing. Cambridge: Polity Press. (2013)

Thane, P. Demographic futures. London: British Academy Policy Centre. (2012)

References

1 **House of Lords**. Ready for ageing? Report. Select Committee on Public Service and Demographic Change. Report of Session 2012–14. HL Paper 140. London: The Stationery Office Limited; 2013.

2 **Thane P**. Demographic futures: new paradigms in public policy. London: British Academy Policy Centre; 2012.

3 **Brocklehurst J**. Geriatric medicine in Britain—the growth of a specialty. Age Ageing. 1997;**26–S4**:5–8.

4 **Barton A, Mulley G**. History of the development of geriatric medicine in the UK. Postgrad Med J. 2003;**79**:229–34.

5 **Carboni D**. Geriatric medicine in the United States and United Kingdom. New York: Greenwood Press; 1982.

6 **Thompson AP**. Problems of ageing and chronic sickness. BMJ. 1949 Jul 30:243–50.

7 **Rowntree S**. Old people: report of a survey committee on the problems of ageing and the care of older people. London: Nuffield Foundation; 1947.

8 **Phillips Report**. Report of the committee on the economic and financial problems of the provision for old age. London: HMSO; 1954.

9 **Sheldon J**. The social medicine of old age. London: Nuffield Foundation; 1948.

10 **Isaacs B, Livingstone M, Neville Y**. Survival of the unfittest. London: Routledge & Kegan Paul; 1972.

11 **Anderson WF, Cowan, NR**. A consultative health centre for older people. Lancet. 1955;**2** 239–40.

12 **Williamson J, Stokoe IH, Gray S, Fisher M, Smith H, McGhee A, Stephenson E**. Old people at home: their unreported needs. Lancet. 1964;**1**:1117–20.

13 **Barrett A, Savva G, Timonen V, Kenny RA**. Fifty plus in Ireland 2011: first results from the Irish Longitudinal Study on Ageing. Dublin: Trinity College; 2011.

14 **Townsend P**. The family life of old people. London: Routledge & Kegan Paul; 1957.

15 **Townsend P**. The last refuge. London: Routledge & Kegan Paul; 1962.

16 **Tunstall J**. Old and alone: a sociological study of old people. London: Routledge and Kegan Paul; 1963.

17 **Felstein I**. Later life: geriatrics today and tomorrow. London: Croom Helm; 1969.

18 **Leonard JC**. Can geriatrics survive? BMJ. 1976;**1**:1335–36.

19 **Townsend P**. The structured dependency of the elderly: a creation of social policy in the twentieth century. Ageing Soc. 1981;**1**:5–28.

20 **Phillipson C**. Reconstructing old age. London: SAGE Books; 1998.

21 **Phillipson C**. Ageing. Cambridge: Polity Press; 2013.

22 **Estes C**. The aging enterprise. San Francisco: Jossey-Bass; 1979.

23 **Twigg, J**. The body in health and social care. London: Palgrave; 2006.

24 **Gilleard C, Higgs P**. Ageing, corporeality and embodiment. London: Anthem Press; 2013.

25 **Davis J, Tallis R**. NHS SOS: how the NHS was betrayed—and how we can save it. London: Oneworld; 2013. Accessed 2 Sep 2013.

26 **Börsch-Supan A, Brandt M, Litwin H, Weber, G, eds**. Active ageing and solidarity between generations in Europe. Berlin: De Gruyter; 2013.

27 **Timonen V, Scharf T, Conlon C, Carney G**. Intergenerational solidarity and justice: towards a new national dialogue. J Intergen Rel. 2012;**10**(3):317–21.

28 **Carstensen L, Fried LP**. The meaning of old age. Submission to Senate Committee on Aging, Washington, DC; nd.

29 **World Health Organization**. Global age friendly cities: a guide. Geneva: WHO; 2007. Accessed 2 Jul 2013. http.://www.who.int/ageing/publications/Global_age_friendly_cities_Guide_English.pdf

30 **Buffel T, Phillipson C, Scharf T**. Experiences of neighbourhood exclusion and inclusion among older people living in deprived inner-city areas in Belgium and England. Ageing Soc. 2013;**33**(1):89–109.

31 **Scharlach A, Lehning A**. Ageing-friendly communities and social inclusion in the United States of America. Ageing Soc. 2013;**33**(1):110–36.

32 **Dublin Declaration on Age-Friendly Cities and Communities in Europe**. 2013. http:// agefriendlycounties.com/images/uploads/downloads/Dublin_Declaration_2013.pdf

33 **Pahl R**. On friendship. Cambridge: Polity Press; 2000.

34 **Marmot M, Allen J, Goldblatt P, Boyce T, McNeish D, Grady M, Geddes I**. Fair society, healthy lives. London: The Marmot Review; 2010.

35 **Office for National Statistics**. Life expectancy at birth and at age 65 by local areas in the United Kingdom, 2004–6 to 2008–10. 2011. Accessed 5 Sep 2013. http://www.ons.gov. uk/ons/publications/all-releases.html?definition=tcm%3A77-22483

36 **Kendig H, Browning C**. A social view on healthy ageing: multi-disciplinary perspectives and Australian evidence. In: Dannefer D, Phillipson C, eds. The SAGE handbook of social gerontology. London: SAGE; 2010. p. 459–71.

37 **Dannefer D, Kelly-Moore J**. Theorizing the life course: new twists in the paths. In: Bengtson V, Gans D, Putney N, Silverstein M, eds. Handbook of theories of aging, 2nd ed. New York: Springer; 2009. p. 389–412.

38 **Le Couteur D, Doust J, Creasey H, Brayne C**. Political drive to screen for pre-dementia: not evidence based and ignores the harms of diagnosis. BMJ.2013;**347**:f5125.

39 **Whitehouse P**. (2007) The next 100 years of Alzheimer's—learning to care not cure. Dementia. 2007;**6**(4):459–62.

40 **O'Neill D**. Am I a gerontologist or a geriatrician. J Am Geriatr Soc. 2012;**60**:1361–3.

Chapter 3

Health and social care services for older people: achievements, challenges, and future directions

Roger Beech

Key points

- The ageing of the population will increase patient demands for acute hospital beds, a scarce and expensive resource.
- Health and social care service options delivered 'closer to home' can improve patient care and reduce older people's demands for acute hospital beds by preventing acute events and providing an alternative.
- The growth of such service options has created a more complex health and social care landscape.
- Therefore, to improve the patient experience and to ensure their timely access to appropriate care, innovations for improving the integration of services for health and social care need to be developed and evaluated.
- Further increasing the evidence base about care closer-to-home service options and ways of improving their integration represents a shared agenda for service commissioners, providers, and academics.

1 Introduction

As a means of responding to the ageing of the population and reducing patient demands for acute hospital care, recent years have seen an expansion of service options for delivering health and social care in the community or at the interface between acute hospital and community-based care. The first part of this chapter discusses the rationale for these service reforms, the types of 'closer-to-home' services that have been introduced, and existing research evidence to support their use. The second part of the chapter moves to a discussion of the current policy drive of encouraging the introduction of initiatives and innovations to achieve a greater integration of services for health and social care. Again the rationale for such developments is discussed, together with the different ways in which this strategy of service integration is being pursued, and existing research evidence about the merits of service changes. Both parts of the chapter expose the need for further research to support the development and evaluation of new services for health and social care. The chapter concludes by highlighting ways in which health and social care staff and researchers must now work together on this agenda of service reform and evaluation in order to achieve the goal of improved health and social care services for older people.

2 An expansion of health and social care services for older people closer to home

2.1 Rationale for service changes

The population of England is ageing (Box 3.1), a fact that will lead to an ongoing rise in demand for services for health and social care. The effects of this demographic change first generated widespread concern towards the end of the 1990s when individuals faced difficulties in obtaining services for unplanned acute inpatient care, particularly during winter months (2).

Box 3.1 The ageing of England's population

- England, in common with most Western states, is facing a rise in the age of its population.
- In comparison to the year 2010, by 2030 there will be 51% more people aged over 65 and 101% aged over 85.
- By 2018, relative to 2008, 50% more individuals will be living with three or more long-term conditions (1).

Drawing on research that estimated that approximately 20% of acute bed use by older people was 'avoidable' (3), the national beds inquiry argued that the way to reduce demands for acute hospital beds was to offer alternative care options that delivered care in patient's homes or other non-acute settings. This policy of developing and expanding care options closer to home was endorsed by subsequent policy documents including the NHS Plan (4) and the National Service Framework for Older People (5). As a result, there has been a growth of care closer-to-home services, often delivered by teams of health and social care staff, which aim to reduce or delay older people's demands for high-cost services such as acute care (Box 3.2).

Box 3.2 Aims of care 'closer-to-home' services

- preventing older people experiencing events that might require acute hospital care (e.g. falls prevention schemes (6)) and schemes to provide more proactive care for older people with long-term conditions (7,8)

- providing an alternative to acute hospital admission or attendance (e.g. rapid response teams (9,10) and hospital-at-home schemes (11) for individuals who experience acute events

- reducing the lengths of stay of patients who require an emergency admission (e.g. residential intermediate care schemes (12) and early supported discharge schemes (13)).

2.2 Research evidence about the impacts of care closer-to-home services

Research studies have investigated the impacts of care closer-to-home schemes on the health of older people and their use of acute hospital services. Randomized controlled trials and/or systematic reviews of randomized controlled trials are regarded as providing the most reliable source of evidence.

Evidence about the impacts of schemes that aim to prevent hospital admissions is somewhat mixed. A systematic review commissioned by the World Health Organization found that falls-prevention schemes, such as multifactorial falls programmes, can reduce an individual's risk of falling, acute events (such as hip fracture), and the associated use of health care resources (14). A systematic review by Shepperd et al. (11) concluded that preventing hospital admissions through the use of hospital-at-home schemes does not adversely affect health outcomes and that patients prefer home care. They also found that hospital-at-home care can be less costly than hospital-based care. However, an evidence review by Purdy (15) found that other than for people with mental health problems, proactively case managing people with long-term conditions does not reduce hospital admissions.

Results from individual trials demonstrate that early-discharge schemes can provide an effective and cost-effective alternative to an extended stay in an acute hospital for patients admitted for conditions such as stroke and chronic obstructive pulmonary disease (COPD) (11,16). A systematic review by Shepperd et al. (17) also found that early-discharge schemes did not have an adverse effect on health outcomes, but the claim that they result in cost savings was questioned. However, this review argued that patients may prefer to have their care delivered in their home.

3 Integrating health and social care services for older people

3.1 Rationale for service changes

While recent developments have increased the options available for patient care, they have also created a more complex landscape for patients and staff to navigate because care closer-to-home-type services are delivered by staff from different disciplines working in different organizations and settings (Box 3.3). Research studies have examined the extent to which patients, such as those with COPD, currently obtain timely and 'seamless' access to needed services for health and social care.

Box 3.3 A more complex health and social care landscape

- Care options available for a person with COPD include those for
  - initial diagnosis and ongoing management (from primary care staff); smoking cessation (from public health teams);
  - 'step-up' care following an exacerbation (from community nursing teams and/or acute hospital staff);
  - pulmonary rehabilitation (from community-based nurses and therapists);
  - end-of-life care (from hospital and hospice staff).
- A person's need for such services will also change over time as they experience gradual or sudden changes in their health status.

A recent study examined the delivery of front-line services received by patients in response to a health crisis that resulted in a 999 call and/or an emergency attendance at an acute hospital (18). Interviews with patients, carers, and staff were used to explore the coordination of services received by patients prior to a health crisis, immediately following the health crisis, and during the ongoing rehabilitation phase. The study found examples of good practice but problems surrounding the delivery of services were evident.

There was underuse of services for preventing health crises. In part this was due to individuals' being slow to access care, or having difficulties in accessing care, following accidents such as a fall or when they felt unwell. In addition, health professionals, such as GPs and staff working in Accident and Emergency Departments, often failed to refer patients to preventative services. For example, frequent fallers were not always directed to falls-prevention services. At the time of a health crisis, there was underuse of services for preventing hospital admissions. This was due to a lack of knowledge about the existence and nature of care closer-to-home services among staff that provided immediate care for patients following a crisis. Finally, during the ongoing rehabilitation phase, communication difficulties between health and social care staff, particularly those working in different organizations and settings, led to a poor patient experience and delays in them gaining timely access to services for ongoing care.

Research elsewhere has generated similar findings. For example, studies by McLeod et al. (19) and Toscan et al. (20,21) have examined care for patients following hip fractures. Both found that communication problems between staff working in different settings led to a poor patient experience and delays in the delivery of care. Reports by the NHS Future Forum and Age UK have also stressed that efforts to improve the integration of health and social care services for older people are now needed as a means of improving patient experience and ensuring that they obtain timely access to appropriate care (22,23).

3.2 Research evidence about the impacts of service integration strategies

Strategies and schemes that aim to achieve a more integrated approach to the delivery of care can take place at different levels in organizations as depicted in Figure 3.1.

At the patient–practitioner interface level, case-management approaches are usually supported by the use of risk stratification tools for identifying individuals who are frequent users of acute hospital services. Typically, these are older patients with complex health and/or social care needs (26).

Such an array of schemes and strategies can create confusion about what is meant by integrated care. Lloyd and Waite (27) define integrated care as

> Care which imposes the patient's perspective as the organizing principle of service delivery and makes redundant old supply-driven models of care provision. Integrated care enables health and social care provision that is flexible, personalized and seamless.

This definition is helpful as it demonstrates that any approach to improve the integration of care should be driven by the needs of patients. Success should also be measured in terms of the extent to which the approach actually achieves or promotes better patient care.

Evidence is still emerging about the ways in which service changes that aim to promote more integrated care affect patient care and the use of resources for health and social care. Research findings to date indicate that although changes

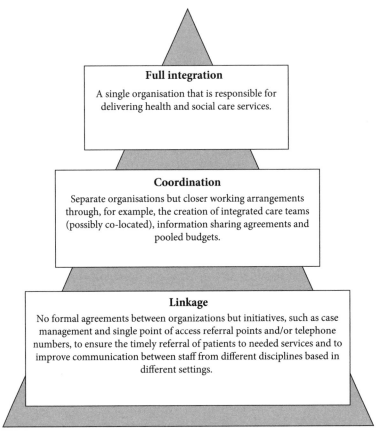

Fig. 3.1 Levels of health and social care service integration.
Adapted from Wistow et al. (24) and Shaw et al. (25).

at the organization level might be necessary to provide leadership and backing for measures to promote more integrated care, they do not of themselves lead to improved care at the patient–practitioner interface (18,28). This is because they need to be accompanied by initiatives to ensure that organizational goals influence the actions of front-line staff.

Emergent findings in relation to the introduction of integrated health and social care teams and the use of case management are more positive. Studies, including evaluations of the English Integrated Care Pilots, have found that these interventions can lead to improved health outcomes for patients and increased satisfaction with care delivery processes among patients, carers, and health and social care staff (26). However, evidence about the impact of such schemes on the overall costs of delivering health and social care remains inconclusive. Indeed, it has been found that case management can lead to an increase in emergency admissions; a possible explanation is that staff are more aware of the needs of their patients (26). The previously cited review by Purdy (15) also raised doubts about the ability of case-management schemes to reduce hospital admissions.

4 Building the evidence base for integrated health and social care services

Although it is increasing, the evidence base to support the introduction of care options closer to home, and for improving their integration, is currently inconclusive (28). This chapter therefore concludes by proposing some principles that health and social care staff and researchers can use to build the evidence base about service changes. These principles draw on guidance produced by the Nuffield Trust, the Medical Research Council, and the approaches that have been used to evaluate the English Integrated Care Pilots (29–31).

4.1 Identify the patient group to be targeted

The development of integrated care schemes and strategies must be driven by the needs of patients. Hence, the first step is to identify those patient groups that are thought to be in need of a more integrated approach to the delivery of care. These patient groups might be individuals suffering from a specific condition, such as COPD, whose care involves inputs from staff with different disciplinary backgrounds working in different settings (Box 3.3). Typically, though, the patient group will cover elderly patients with multimorbidity and/or with complex social care needs (26).

4.2 Clarify why this patient group needs a more integrated approach to the delivery of care

Patients and staff not accessing relevant services or not accessing them in a timely manner is a key driver for the development of integrated care (22,23). Baseline analysis could be used to identify the types of evidence-based services that are not being accessed efficiently. Also, it may be important to develop an understanding of why they are not being accessed and how poor integration of care is affecting the health of patients, their experiences of health and social care, and their use of services for health and social care.

4.3 Use baseline analysis to inform the design of new interventions

The previous step ensures that schemes and strategies for promoting more integrated care are driven by an understanding of the problems that are affecting the delivery of services and how these impact patient care. This step involves the development of a theory about why a new intervention might overcome current problems. Hence a decision to co-locate staff or to create integrated care teams, for example, would be made because this is seen as the best way of addressing current service delivery problems.

4.4 Adopt a theory of change design to evaluate the impacts of new interventions

Integrated care is an enabler because it involves putting in place systems and processes that aim to ensure that patients obtain access to relevant services. Hence evaluation activity needs to focus on care delivery processes as well as impact on patients. The evaluation framework used should be underpinned by the theory that was developed to support the design of an intervention. For example, if the intervention is seen as a means of improving communication and information sharing between staff, changes in these domains would need to be monitored (process evaluation). The reasons for any residual difficulties would also be explored. The impact evaluation would be linked to the ways in which the intervention was seen as generating benefits for patients. For example, a reduction in falls and the consequences of falls would be monitored if the intervention aimed to ensure that more individuals who were at risk of falls were referred to a falls-prevention scheme. The ways in which the intervention affects patients' use of resources for health and social care is also likely to be a key component of the impact evaluation.

The authors of the review by the Nuffield Trust (29) recognize that the complex nature of interventions to improve the integration of services for health and social care means that their introduction and refinement takes time. This has implications for the precise focus and methods that will be used to support the evaluation. When a new intervention is first introduced, the monitoring of process evaluation issues might be more important. Once the nature of the intervention has become more established, more rigorous evaluation designs and a greater focus upon the impacts of new schemes may be more appropriate (29,30).

4.5 Use evaluation findings to guide needed service modifications and to reinforce the need for service integration

There should be ongoing feedback of emergent evaluation findings. Results from the evaluation of care delivery processes will allow strategies to resolve residual difficulties to be put in place. Findings from the evaluation of impacts for patients and staff can also help to engineer ongoing support for new integrated care interventions from health and social care staff. This is important as these interventions usually involve health and social care staff working in new ways.

5 Conclusion

In the current climate of financial constraints, the inconclusive evidence about the financial merit of schemes and strategies for promoting more integrated and community-based services for delivering health and social care might act as a barrier to their continued development. However, it is important that this agenda of service development and evaluation continues. If not, the current problems surrounding the delivery of health and social care services will remain with patients having poor care experiences and problems in accessing relevant services.

Key guidelines, policy documents, reviews, and websites relevant to this chapter

The key current sources of information such as websites and policy documents are already referenced within the chapter. However, this is a rapidly evolving area. Useful websites to monitor are:

The King's Fund. Integrated care: making it happen.

<http://www.kingsfund.org.uk/>

The Nuffield Trust. From the blog: latest expert analysis.

<http://www.nuffieldtrust.org.uk/>

The Department of Health.

<https://www.gov.uk/government/organisations/department-of-health>

National Institute for Health and Clinical Evidence.

<http://www.nice.org.uk>

Cochrane Summaries.

<http://summaries.cochrane.org>

References

1 **Select Committee on Public Service and Demographic Change—First Report.** Ready for ageing? London: Parliament; 2013. Accessed 30 Jul 2013. http://www.publications.parliament.uk/pa/ld201213/ldselect/ldpublic/140/14002.htm

2 **Beech R.** Evidence on effectiveness of intermediate care. In: Roe B, Beech R, eds. Intermediate and continuing care: policy and practice. Oxford: Blackwell; 2005. p. 106–118.

3 **McDonagh MS, Smith D, Goddard M.** Measuring appropriate use of acute beds: a systematic review of methods and results. Health Policy. 2000;**53**:157–84.

4 **Department of Health.** The NHS Plan: a plan for investment, a plan for reform. London: Department of Health; 2000. Accessed 30 Jul 2013. http://www.dh.gov.uk/en/ Publicationsandstatistics/Publications/PublicationsPolicyAndGuidance/DH_4002960

5 **Department of Health.** National service framework for older people. London: Department of Health; 2001. Accessed 30 Jul 2013. https://www.gov.uk/government/ uploads/system/uploads/attachment_data/file/198033/National_Service_Framework_ for_Older_People.pdf

6 **Beech R, DeVilliers R, Thorniley-Jones H, Welch H, Douglas C, Roe B, Russell W, Russell M.** Promoting evidence informed service development: a study of falls services in Cheshire. Primary Health Care Res Develop. 2010;**11**(3):222–32.

7 **Russell M, Roe B, Beech R, Russell W.** Service developments for managing people with long term conditions using case management approaches: an example from the UK. Int J Integr Care. 2009 Feb 23;9. Accessed 5 Sep 2012. http://www.ijic.org/index.php/ijic/ article/view/303/605

8 **Sheaff R, Boaden R, Sargent P, Pickard S, Gravelle H, Parker S, Roland M.** Impacts of case management for frail elderly people: a qualitative study. J Health Serv Res Pol. 2009;**14**(2):88–95.

9 **Stevenson J, Spencer L.** Developing intermediate care: a guide for health and social services professionals. London: The Kings Fund; 2002.

10 **Beech R, Russell W, Little R, Sherlow S.** An evaluation of a multidisciplinary team for intermediate care at home. Int J Integr Care. 2004 Oct-Dec 4. Accessed 5 Sep 2012. http://www.ijic.org/index.php/ijic/article/view/113/226

11 **Shepperd S, Doll H, Angus RM, Clarke MJ, Iliffe S, Kalra L, Ricauda NA, Wilson AD.** 'Hospital at home' services to avoid admission to hospital. The Cochrane Library; 2011. Accessed 24 Jul 2013. http://summaries.cochrane.org/CD007491/hospital-at-home- services-to-avoid-admission-to-hospital

12 **Young J.** The evidence base for intermediate care. Geriatr Med. 2002;**32**(10):11–4.

13 **Beech R, Rudd AG, Tilling K, Wolfe CDA.** Economic consequences of early inpatient discharge to community based rehabilitation for stroke in an inner-London teaching hospital. Stroke. 1999;**30**(4):729–35.

14 **Todd C, Skelton D.** What are the main risk factors for falls among older people and what are the most effective interventions to prevent these falls? Copenhagen: WHO Regional Office for Europe (Health Evidence Network report); 2004. Accessed 29 Jul 2013. http://www.euro.who.int/__data/assets/pdf_file/0018/74700/E82552.pdf

15 **Purdy S.** Avoiding hospital admissions: what does the research evidence say? London: The King's Fund; 2010. Accessed 30 Jul 2013. http://www.kingsfund.org.uk/publications/ avoiding-hospital-admissions

16 **NICE.** Commissioning an assisted-discharge service for patients with COPD. National Institute for Health and Care Excellence; 2009. Accessed 30 Jul 2013. http://www.nice. org.uk/usingguidance/commissioningguides/assdissvcpatientscopd/ commissioninganassisteddischargeservice.jsp

17 Shepperd S, Doll H, Broad J, Gladman J, Iliffe S, Langhorne P, Richards S, Martin F, Harris R. Services for patients discharged home early. Cochrane Collaboration; 2011. Accessed 24 Jul 2013. http://summaries.cochrane.org/CD000356/services-for-patients-discharged-home-early

18 Beech R, Henderson C, Ashby S, Dickinson A, Sheaff R, Windle K, Wistow G, Knapp M. Does integrated governance lead to integrated patient care? Health Soc Care Comm. 2013 Nov;21(6):598–605.

19 McLeod J, McMurray J, Walker JD, Heckman GA, Stolee P. Care transitions for older patients with musculoskeletal disorders: continuity from the providers' perspective. Int J Integr Care. 2011 Apr 18;11. Accessed 30 Jul 2013. http://www.ijic.org/index.php/ijic/article/view/555/1240

20 Toscan J, Mairs K, Hinton S, Stolee P. Integrated transitional care: patient, informal caregiver and health care provider perspectives on care transitions for older people with hip fracture. Int J Integr Care. 2012 Apr 13;12. Accessed 30 Jul 2013. http://www.ijic.org/index.php/ijic/article/view/URN%3ANBN%3ANL%3AUI%3A10-1-112878/1531

21 Toscan J, Manderson B, Sant SM, Stolee P. 'Just another fish in the pond': the transitional care experience of a hip fracture patient. Int J Integr Care. 2013 Apr-Jun;13. Accessed 30 Jul 2013. http://www.ijic.org/index.php/ijic/article/view/URN%3ANBN%3ANL%3AUI%3A10-1-114597/2017

22 Age UK. Agenda for later life 2012. Policy priorities for active ageing. Age UK; 2012. Accessed 30 Jul 2013. http://www.ageuk.org.uk/Global/AgendaforLaterLifeReport2012.pdf?dtrk=true

23 NHS Future Forum. Integration: a report from the NHS Future Forum. NHS Future Forum; 2012. Accessed 30 Jul 2013. https://www.gov.uk/government/uploads/system/uploads/attachment_data/file/216425/dh_132023.pdf

24 Wistow G, Waddington E, Kitt I. Commissioning care closer to home: final report. London: Association of Directors of Adult Social Services; 2010. Accessed 30 Jul 2013. http://www.adass.org.uk/AdassMedia/stories/Publications/Commissioning%20care_Layout%202.pdf

25 Shaw S, Rosen R, Rumbold B. An overview of integrated care in the NHS. What is integrated care? London: Nuffield Trust; 2011. Accessed 30 Jul 2013. http://www.nuffieldtrust.org.uk/sites/files/nuffield/publication/what_is_integrated_care_research_report_june11_0.pdf

26 Roland M, Lewis R, Steventon A, Abel G, Adams J, Bardsley M, Brereton L, Chitnis X, Conklin A, Staetsky L, Tunkel S, Ling T. Case management for at-risk elderly patients in the English integrated care pilots: observational study of staff and patient experience and secondary care utilisation. Int J Integr Care. 2012 Jul 24;12. Accessed 30 Jul 2013. http://www.ijic.org/index.php/ijic/article/view/URN%3ANBN%3ANL%3AUI%3A10-1-113731/1772

27 Lloyd J, Wait S. Integrated care: a guide for policy makers. London: Alliance for Health and the Future; 2005.

28 Ling T, Brereton L, Conklin A, Newbould J, Roland M. Barriers and facilitators to integrated care: experiences from the English integrated care pilots. Int J Integr Care. 2012 Jul 24;12. Accessed 30 Jul 2013. http://www.ijic.org/index.php/ijic/article/view/URN%3ANBN%3ANL%3AUI%3A10-1-113730/1770

29 **Bardsley M, Steventon A, Smith J, Dixon J**. Evaluating integrated and community-based care: how do we know what works? London: Nuffield Trust; 2013. Accessed 30 Jul 2013. http://www.nuffieldtrust.org.uk/sites/files/nuffield/publication/evaluation_summary_final.pdf

30 **Medical Research Council**. Developing and evaluating complex interventions: new guidance. London: MRC; 2008. Accessed 30 Jul 2013. http://www.mrc.ac.uk/Utilities/Documentrecord/index.htm?d=MRC004871

31 **Ling T, Bardsley M, Adams J, Lewis R, Roland M**. Evaluation of UK integrated care pilots: research protocol. Int J Integr Care. 2010 Sep 27;10. Accessed 30 Jul 2013. http://www.ijic.org/index.php/ijic/article/view/URN%3ANBN%3ANL%3AUI%3A10-1-100969/1069

Chapter 4

Service models

Finbarr C Martin

Key points

- There is increasing concern about quality of care received by older people in our health services.

- Real progress over recent decades in overcoming ignorance and ageism is at risk if these services cannot become age-attuned.

- Today's older people are older, more numerous, and present complex challenges of multimorbidity and frailty.

- Traditional divisions of staff and skills between primary and secondary care, and between clinical specialties, are an obstacle to meeting the challenge.

- Promising innovative new models of care are emerging and will need refinement through research and experience.

- Skills and attitudes needed to recognize and manage the geriatric syndromes must be mainstreamed through education, training, and dissemination of good practice.

- Specialists in old-age medicine and mental health cannot do it all, but must champion this transformation.

1 Introduction

An ageing society represents a real success but brings new challenges to health and social care provision. In recent years, there has been a deluge of press reports, inquiries, and political attention to the plight of older people in the health and social care services. Increasing concern about quality of care for older people is welcome. Unfortunately it is often couched in negative terms of a 'tsunami' of demand and moral panic on loss of caring capacity of staff.

In truth, there has never been a golden age of health services for older people. The models of care which cope reasonably well with acute episodic illness in previously well adults do not do well with the multimorbidity and frailty of old age which this chapter will briefly describe. Getting services right is a continuous process of adaption—to new circumstances, new cohorts of older people, and the ever-changing possibilities of medicine and health care. Making sense of current services and their attendant challenges is as much an exercise in political history as it is in medical history. And going forward successfully will depend as much on appreciating the social and cultural perspective as on new innovations in treatment.

Specialists in old-age health care, including geriatricians and old-age psychiatrists, need to be in the vanguard of getting health services fit for our modern population's needs: in short we need an age-attuned NHS. This will include new models of specialist services but also embedding the necessary attitudes, skills, and know-how throughout the service.

2 Towards a strategic approach to older people

The 1980s saw a reduction in the scope and a shrinkage in the size of specialist older peoples' medical services with the welcome development of acute wards on general hospital sites but the almost total closure of NHS long-stay facilities and a significant reduction of designated rehabilitation wards. Facility to admit older people directly gave geriatricians an increasing role in their acute medical care. But pressures of beds and reductions of doctors' working time forced amalgamation into all-age adult medical admission wards, with geriatricians playing a larger role generally but at the expense of their time commitment to more specialized old-age services.

On the positive side, geriatricians' presence on the acute hospital site and better access for older people to higher-tech medicine resulted in many developing subspecialty skills and roles: e.g. in stroke, cardiorespiratory conditions, and orthogeriatrics.

Hospital bed numbers reduced with dramatic reductions in lengths of hospital stay outstripping the gradual increase in numbers of emergency and planned admissions. *The NHS Plan 2000* (1) made continuing reduction of acute beds official policy, investing great hope in the capacity of community services to accommodate increasing complexity and volume of need. The large reduction in total medical and geriatric beds was accompanied by growth of alternative community-based services used mainly by older people, and featuring various degrees of health and social care collaboration.

Collectively these are known as *intermediate care* (IC) as they address the care phase between medical recovery and functional stability, with the general strategic aim of reducing hospital use while attempting to promote independence and avoid unnecessary dependence on institutional or domiciliary social care. The word *intermediate* also highlights that these service models were distinct both from hospitals and primary care. Geriatricians have rarely been in a clear-cut leadership role. Examples are described throughout in relation to alternatives to hospital admission and to post-acute care.

The *National Service Framework* (NSF) for older people in 2001 (2) set out for the first time a government view of the scope of services for older people with some clarification of the role of specialists. The NSF was organized around geriatric syndromes such as falls rather than organ-based conditions. This supported the emergence of more evidence-based service models.

3 The changing nature of health in old age

Health and social care use are concentrated at the beginning and towards the end of life. When the NHS was founded, over a third of the population died before age 65. Half a century later, it had fallen to approximately 18% and the chance of surviving from birth to age 85 has more than doubled for men over the last three decades from 14% in 1980–1982 to 38% in 2009–2011. Most of us will die in relative old age, but that age is getting older, as survival within older age is increasing rapidly. Life expectancy at age 65 in England and Wales for men in 2009–2011 rose by 5.1 years since 1980–1982 when it was 13.0 years. Women have seen a smaller increase of 3.8 years since 1980–1982 when it was 17.0 years (3). 'Thus 'older people' are older and more numerous than they were, but they are also different, and the nature of this difference is central to appreciating the way that services need to change.

The number of people living with one or more long-term medical conditions (LTCs) is increasing: 40% of those 65+ report two or more self-reported LTCs. But this does not justify a gloomy outlook (4). Rates of LTCs do correlate generally with poorer well-being, but neither the English Longitudinal Study of Ageing (5) nor the Census (4) show post-65 rates of poor health or disability to be increasing. Indeed, the Health Survey for England (6) shows that mental well-being peaks at ages 65–74. But rates do increase—most people age 75+ report three or more LTCs—and LTCs have increasing impact. LTCs account for 55% of GP appointments, 77% of in-patient bed days, and approximately 70% of Englands total health budget (7).

But the most profound difference characterizing health care in older ages is the presence of frailty. This can be defined in several ways, with prevalence varying accordingly from 6% upwards (8). It results from the effects of ageing, lifestyle, events, and disease combining to render bodily and mental functions impaired, with the resultant diminished reserve making the individual vulnerable to decompensation with additional 'minor' illnesses or challenges. This lost resilience may manifest as the geriatric syndromes of falls, immobility, confusion, and a general failure to thrive or to recover from new illness (9). It is strongly associated with poor outcomes, increased mortality, and use of health and social care (10, 11).

3.1 The implications for evidence-based medicine

LTCs emerging in later life include osteoporosis, with the risk of fractures; urinary incontinence, which affects a quarter of women over 65; and dementia. But conditions of frailer older people are significantly less well managed in primary care than the familiar middle-age conditions of hypertension, diabetes, and respiratory disease (12), even when national clinical guidance exists, such as for secondary falls and fractures prevention (13–15). Furthermore, while the presence of several LTCs is the reality, clinical guidance is generally arranged around single conditions, and the research providing the evidence for this guidance has often excluded co-morbidity or frailty (16, 17).

Clinical decision making is more difficult in the presence of co-morbidities and frailty. Attribution of risk from individual components of a complex mix of conditions is difficult. Estimating potential benefit in terms of ameliorating symptoms, disability, or mortality risk is also difficult; indeed the relative importance of these differs between individuals and at different stages of life. Nowhere is this more pressing than for the most complex patients who are residents of care homes. We need new evidence reflecting these complexities. Addressing these issues is a challenge both to primary care and specialist geriatric services.

3.2 Health policies and levers

Centralized targets have galvanized sluggish processes without much impact on quality. Financial incentives have improved care quality of some LTC management in primary care and in several hospital services. Clinically led networks and other professional drivers have had greater impact. It remains to be seen whether clinically led commissioning will improve or impede the integration of services which is so important for frail older people.

Considerable funding and managerial effort has gone into short-term initiatives to reduce the rate of acute hospital admissions of older people, usually based on weak or nonexistent evidence. Most have clear strategic aims but ill-defined clinical content and are delivered by undertrained staff. They have failed to grasp the complexities outlined above and little has been achieved (18).

In contrast, evidence is growing for new service models built on the technology of comprehensive geriatric assessment (CGA) (19).

4 Current and emerging models of care

Since older people are the majority of health services users, health-care providers with specialist expertise need to be more numerous. The geriatrician-led multidisciplinary team (MDT) should provide much of the direct clinical care in hospitals for the more complex and frail medically ill older patients. But they also need to support embedding appropriate clinical approaches in the wider hospital and community health services. This implies transforming services, education, and training of the general health workforce and supporting the clinical care of older patients provided by other secondary care specialists, physicians, and surgeons. The following sections describe these roles within clinical contexts.

4.1 Acute and episodic illness

Involvement of members of the geriatric MDT at the 'front door' of the acute hospital is becoming more common, notably occupational therapists, physiotherapists, and geriatricians. There is increasing evidence that re-attendance of older patients to the emergency department (ED) is predictable by relatively simple assessment at the index visit. This has been linked to various service initiatives aimed at reducing this risk.

4.1.1 Interface geriatrics

This term has emerged to denote the need both for the right clinical skills and the right connectivity between the hospital and the community. Services described so far provide a range of clinical and social-care responses, and significant impact is claimed by evaluations which do not yet constitute Class I evidence (20). A recent randomized controlled trial (RCT) showed that it is feasible to apply CGA with frail older people in the ED and this was associated with reduced admissions and readmissions (21). This is promising, but complex interventions of this nature are likely highly context dependent in effectiveness and cost, and there may be no generalizable elements except general clinical principles.

Case finding in urgent-care settings usually includes links to less specialized community-based IC teams with a focus on hospital admission avoidance. The Cochrane Review of such services (22) summarized with a meta-analysis the findings from ten RCTs, only three of which included older patients with mix of conditions, one from England. Overall no differences in mortality or other outcomes such as functional ability, quality of life, or cognitive ability were found. Patients reported increased satisfaction with admission avoidance ('hospital at home'). The settings, services, and patients were so variable that no practically useful conclusions can be drawn. Nevertheless such services now exist in almost all local health services in England and many elsewhere in UK. There are therefore plenty of questions to be addressed by future clinical and health services research:

- Can a brief CGA be embedded into routine ED assessments of older people to identify those for whom a more time-consuming specialized approach is worthwhile?

- What clinical features predict a better recovery of function by receiving home-based rather than hospital-based care? This will need reliable methods to operationalize relevant psychosocial aspects such as self-efficacy.

- Can telehealth be developed to enable remote diagnostic assessment of patients presenting acutely but with nonspecific 'geriatric syndromes' sufficiently reliably to safely limit hospital attendances?

- Is it cost-effective to provide home-based care for acutely ill patients as an alternative to hospital admission?

- What skills and training enable teams to function safely and cost-effectively?

ED attendance also offers an opportunity for case finding linked to secondary prevention. The evidence of benefit is best established for falls (23), but this trial and others also demonstrated gains in functional independence through a CGA approach to attendees who had fallen. Evidence-based clinical guidance (13) recommends establishing referral pathways from ED or other urgent-care services to falls services but optimal methods to achieve this are not established.

4.1.2 Optimizing early care of acutely ill older patients

During the 1980s and 1990s, direct acute admission to specialist geriatric medical wards from primary care or from EDs was common: there was therefore debate about how best to segment adult admission responsibilities from general medicine—by condition, by age, etc. Most hospitals now have all-age acute medical admission units, so the question is how best to deploy specialist skills as part of an integrated approach. In 2012 geriatricians provided a larger share than any other medical specialty of the medical 'take in' admitting service, but very often even frail complex older people would have no access to the geriatrics MDT if admitted on other days of the week.

The obvious folly of this has resulted in the creation of specialist liaison services: therapists, nurses, and geriatricians are deployed in various combinations to identify key clinical issues, such as geriatric syndromes, using a CGA-based approach. This enables early use of evidence-based approaches to delirium, falls' risk, incontinence, and mobility preservation during the acute phase of illness, and directing suitable patients for ongoing specialist care. There are usually links to community post-acute IC services but also to 'hot' clinics—clinics providing specialist geriatric assessment and treatments.

The evidence base for this liaison approach is still weak (24). But some general principles are reasonably well established from systematic review (25). A systematic review of 22 RCTs evaluating 10,315 participants in six countries (19) found that patients who underwent CGA were more likely to be alive (0.76, 0.64 to 0.90; $p = 0.001$) and in their own homes at median 12 months follow-up compared with patients who received general medical care. They were also 22% less likely to have been admitted to a care home, which has significant financial implications. In general, the impact of the specialist input was associated with the degree of direct clinical involvement rather than advice: effects were greater when the intervention included designated specialist wards.

Future research questions include:

- Can a short screening assessment approach identify patients most likely to benefit?
- What are the characteristics of specialist care that make the difference and can they be transplanted to general wards?

With or without liaison teams, there is a need to embed into acute hospital services evidence-based approaches to the common adverse effects of illness such as delirium (26) and falls (13), although national audits have not yet demonstrated that either have been implemented successfully (27, 28).

4.1.3 Support for frail older people undergoing surgery

Frail older people are at higher risk of adverse outcomes and poor recovery. Co-morbidity rather than age is the best predictor. Traditional pre-operative assessments have focused on cardiorespiratory aspects of safety for anaesthesia. A CGA approach can augment this with gains in clinical outcomes and resources use (29). Although this approach has face validity, and is spreading through the English NHS, the evidence base remains weak. The main processes included in such services are:

- refining risk assessment to enable better risk/benefit estimation
- pre-operative medical and functional optimization, anticipating the entire patient pathway back to functional independence at home
- peri-operative medical care with a particular focus on delirium and mobility.

4.1.4 Orthogeriatric services

Joint working with orthopaedic services on older patients with hip fracture was pioneered by geriatrician Irvine and orthopaedic surgeon Devas (30). The majority of hospitals have some arrangement to provide geriatrician or geriatrics MDT input to post-operative care and rehabilitation. The Cochrane Review summarized results from 13 trials involving 2,498 older, usually female, patients (31). There were trends towards benefit in mortality, functional outcomes, and readmissions, but none reached conventional levels of statistical significance. The trial comparing primarily home-based multidisciplinary rehabilitation with usual inpatient care found marginally improved function, but this was associated with longer periods of rehabilitation and doubtful cost-effectiveness. A later review considered the broader evidence for ongoing rehabilitation to improve mobility function and found insufficient evidence to recommend any specific service model or intervention (32).

In contrast, several RCTs have demonstrated benefits in terms of mortality, delirium, and clinical outcomes associated with a more intense medically oriented approach at the acute stage after fracture (33, 34). An evidence-based model for systematic orthogeriatric care including secondary prevention is set out in a British Orthopaedic Association Blue Book clinical practice guide (35). The model forms the basis for the financial incentive in the best-practice tariff introduced by the Department of Health in England in 2010. It is credited with galvanizing significant improvements in mortality, as well as reductions in hospital lengths of stay and better secondary prevention, all documented by the continuing audits of the National Hip Fracture Database (36).

4.2 Optimizing post-acute recovery

The traditional model of general-hospital-based, designated rehabilitation wards, receiving patients after a period of acute treatment and assessment, has all but disappeared in the UK. No consistent pattern of service model has emerged to take on this function. The traditional model would now be classified as Level 3 in the service model descriptions of the rehabilitation medical specialty (37), characterized by mixed conditions and generic rehabilitation processes. Specialist stroke rehabilitation has consolidated separately with rapid and widespread development of specialist units nationally and internationally, driven by evidence from stroke unit trials (see Chapter 13).

It is likely that the major changes in acute care, such as intensive early investigation and treatments, and discouragement of bed rest, have significantly changed the nature of post-acute care, although the evidence for this is not well documented. Nevertheless at least half of patients have reduced functional ability on hospital discharge compared with before the acute episode (38, 39). The growth of 'prosthetic' social provision has accommodated some of this increased need. Community hospitals are less numerous and have never had a consistent, well-defined service model. One RCT of a model incorporating geriatrician clinical leadership operating in seven hospitals was shown to be safe, with slightly better functional outcomes and comparable costs and patient satisfaction (40). Patients were mostly female, in their mid-80s, living alone, nearly 30% with cognitive impairment, and half with preadmission ADL limitation, transferred about a week after acute admission. Capital costs to create new community hospitals may not appear justified on these findings.

4.2.1 Intermediate care

The more common model is the supported or early discharge type of IC service. Despite national guidance on suitable staffing, casemix, and clinical governance (41), a national audit has shown marked variability in capacity, working methods, resource use, and clinical casemix (42). The Cochrane Review in 2009 (43) presented the results of meta-analyses using individual patient level data where available. There were slightly higher short-term readmission rates for older patients with a mix of conditions but no difference in mortality (relevant as some services incorporated early discharge), and, positively, subsequent institutional care use was lower and satisfaction was higher with IC compared to usual care. Unfortunately, due to heterogeneity, summative research evidence does not clarify the most cost-effective approaches, but well conducted individual trials are helpful as long as their context is understood as an explanatory factor in local effectiveness (44).

The essential first steps in developing IC in any locality are to define the nature of the service level problem that needs solving and to design the referral criteria and clinical processes accordingly, and then to ensure that there are sufficient performance data and clinical governance to keep it on track.

4.3 Management of long-term conditions and frailty

Geriatricians clinically lead many condition-specific services for LTCs, but the prevalent comorbidity and multidimensional nature of patients' needs suggest that the geriatrician alone is rarely sufficient.

4.3.1 Interspecialty collaboration

There is no evidence to guide a specific form of collaborative service. Most involve system specialists and specialist nurses, such as for continence (with urologists and urogynaecologists), movement disorders (neurologists and specialist nurses), and heart failure (cardiologists). There is authoritative clinical guidance in all these areas so that the effectiveness of these services locally can be judged by their performance against standards and this is helped where national audit programmes exist. Feasibility and cost-effectiveness is likely to be context dependent, and this precludes prescriptive statements about service design.

4.3.2 Systematic collaboration with primary care

There is currently a dearth of evidence base for the local protocols for prompting referrals to or to guide follow-up by geriatricians for conditions that are mainly the remit of primary care. An example is in the prevention of falls and fragility fractures, which are associated with osteopaenia or osteoporosis. The NICE guidance referred to does not clarify the precise care pathways as there is no evidence to guide this. Financial incentives for secondary bone health treatments are intended to promote a move towards primary care. Geriatricians' training equip them to play a leading role in planned shared care or care pathways for these and other common syndromes in old age.

4.4 Support for older people in care homes

The move to a care home is a major life event with significant personal and financial consequences. Systematic assessment based on CGA principles reduces premature moves into care homes by optimizing individuals' capabilities and maximizing use of alternative support solutions. Involvement in these local processes is a core responsibility for geriatric medicine specialists.

Residents of care homes have complex health care needs, reflecting multiple long-term conditions, significant disability, and frailty. The social care model is central but insufficient to meet their needs. Indeed, no policy of coordinated health care has been developed to meet these needs, and a number of local models of care have emerged. General practice in many areas does not appear equipped or willing to fill this void unsupported. Availability of relevant health care is highly variable (45). The various services that have arisen to meet perceived need, such as nurse practitioners or care home dedicated GPs, but these initiatives tend not to be sustained beyond project funding and depend on the commitment of local clinical champions (46). There is no Class I evidence to support a specific model, but a summary of the evidence drawn from a mix of methodologies suggests that the following are associated with higher satisfaction of residents and care homes' staff:

- prompt transfer of multidisciplinary assessment clinical information to the care home

◆ determining health care objectives and agreement on advance clinical care plans to reduce unplanned admission to hospital care services and inappropriate interventions at the end of life

◆ nurses working as case managers to augment the contribution of primary care

◆ community pharmacy services supporting medication reviews to improve medication use

◆ input from community mental health teams to reduce inappropriate psychotropics and sedative use

◆ support tools and care frameworks to enable a systematic approach to joint working between care homes, community nursing, and other health professionals.

4.5 **End-of-life care**

Geriatricians and the MDTs that care for inpatients should be clinically competent to provide high quality end-of-life care, but this may be augmented by the use of evidence-based approaches to care planning. Guidance for all hospital-based physicians, including models for anticipatory clinical management, and managing uncertain outcomes (the Amber Care Bundle), have been developed for use in the acute setting (47).

5 **New horizons**

5.1 **Geriatric oncology**

Developments in oncology treatments and changing attitudes of both patients and doctors have resulted in many older people receiving treatments, with the attendant risks of toxicity as well as benefits. Evidence is emerging for the positive role of CGA in guiding treatment decisions. Collaborative working is in its infancy in UK but has been promoted by several Department of Health initiatives. The focus is on embedding brief assessment to flag up frailty and then co-treatment to optimize outcomes. This seems likely to expand.

5.2 **Frailty as a long-term condition**

Despite strong face validity and policy intent, there is little evidence to support systematic care screening among community-dwelling older adults with the intention of early detection and case management. A limitation of attempts so far may reflect the difficulty in identifying frailty (see Chapter 7) rather than co-morbidity. Combining the social and health paradigms in reducing dependency, based on primary-care-based risk assessment remains an attractive option for which the involvement of geriatricians is likely to be helpful.

6 **Conclusion**

In developed and most developing countries, the health care of older people has become the predominant clinical and organizational challenge for the twenty-first century. Improving access and skill in bringing conventional disease-based medicine to older people was the task of the latter half of the last century; incorporating an understanding of ageing and frailty is the next task. Traditional divisions of labour between medicine and surgery and between hospital, community, and primary care are outmoded. New models and approaches are needed. Specialists in old-age medicine and mental health can be champions of this transformation, but they cannot do it all. The attitudes, knowledge, and skills needed for a successful health and social care system in an ageing society must be embedded deeply and widely through education, training, and dissemination of good practice.

Websites relevant to this chapter

<http://www.kingsfund.org.uk/publications/making-our-health-and-care-systems-fit-ageing-population>

<http://summaries.cochrane.org/CD006211/comprehensive-geriatric-assessment-for-older-adults-admitted-to-hospital>

Key guidelines, policy documents, and reviews

The National Service Framework for Older People.

<https://www.gov.uk/government/uploads/system/uploads/attachment_data/file/198033/National_Service_Framework_for_Older_People.pdf>

References

1 **Department of Health**. The NHS Plan: a plan for investment, a plan for reform. Cm 4818-I. London: Stationary Office; 2000.

2 **Department of Health**. National Service Framework: older people. 198033. London: Stationary Office; 2001.

3 **Office for National Statistics**. Interim life tables, England and Wales, 2009–2011. Accessed 16 Sep 2013. http://www.ons.gov.uk/ons/rel/lifetables/interim-life-tables/2009-11/stb-2009-11.html

4 **Office for National Statistics**. 2011 Census for England and Wales. Accessed 11 Sep 2013. http://www.ons.gov.uk/ons/guide-method/census/2011/index.html

5 **UK Data Service 2013.** English Longitudinal Study of Ageing. Accessed 16 Sep 2013. http://ukdataservice.ac.uk/get-data.aspx

6 **Department of Health.** Health Survey for England 2012. Accessed 16 Sep 2013. https:// www.gov.uk/government/publications/health-survey-for-england-2011

7 **Office for National Statistics.** General Household Survey, 2007. Accessed 30 Sep 2013. http://www.ons.gov.uk/ons/rel/ghs/general-household-survey/2007-report/index.html

8 **Rothman M, Leo-Summers L, Gill T Prognostic significance of potential frailty criteria.** J Am Geriatr Soc 2008;**56**(12):2211–6.

9 **Lally F, Crome P.** Understanding frailty. Postgrad Med J. 2007;**83**:16–20.

10 **Fried LP, Tangen CM, Walston J, et al.** Frailty in older adults: evidence for a phenotype. J Gerontol A-Biol. 2001;**56**:M146–56.

11 **Kuh D, Sayer AA, Ben Shlomo Y, et al.** A life-course approach to health aging, frailty and capability. J Gerontol A-Biol. 2007;**62A**:717–21.

12 **Steel N, Bachman M, Maisey S, et al.** Self-reported quality of care consistent with 32 indicators. National population survey of adults aged 50 or more in England. BMJ.2008;**337**:a957.

13 **National Institute for Clinical Excellence.** Falls: the assessment and prevention of falls in older people. Report no. CG21. London: Royal College of Nursing; 2004.

14 **Royal College of Physicians.** National audit of the organisation of services for falls and bone health of older people. London: Royal College of Physicians; 2009.

15. **Royal College of Physicians.** Report of the 2011 inpatient falls pilot audit. Accessed 20 Sep 2013. http://www.rcplondon.ac.uk/sites/default/files/documents/inpatient-falls-final-report-0.pdf

16 **Kings Fund.** The management of people with long term conditions. London: Kings Fund; 2010.

17 **Barnett K, Mercer S, Norbury M, et al.** Epidemiology of multimorbidity and implications for healthcare, research and medical education: a cross-sectional study. Lancet. 2012;**380**(9836):37–43.

18 **Roland M, Abel G.** Reducing emergency admissions: are we on the right track? BMJ. 2012;**345**:e6017.

19 **Ellis G, Whitehead M, Robinson D, et al.** Comprehensive geriatric assessment for older people admitted to hospital: a meta-analysis of randomised controlled trials. BMJ. 2011;**343**:d6553.

20 **PSSRU.** The National Evaluation of Partnerships for Older People Projects: executive summary, 2009. Accessed 16 Sep 2013. http://www.pssru.ac.uk/pdf/rs053.pdf

21 **Conroy SP, Ansari K, Williams M, et al.** A controlled evaluation of comprehensive geriatric assessment in the emergency department: the 'Emergency Frailty Unit'. Age Ageing. 2014;**43**(1):109–114. Epub 2013 Jul 23.

22 **Shepperd S, Doll H, Broad J, et al.** Early discharge hospital at home. Cochrane Database Syst Rev. 2009(1);CD000356. doi: 10.1002/14651858.CD000356.pub3

23 **Close J, Ellis M, Hooper R, Glucksman E, Jackson S, Swift C.** Prevention of falls in the elderly trial (PROFET): a randomised controlled trial. Lancet. 1999;**353**:93–7.

24 **Harari D, Martin FC, Buttery A, O'Neill S, Hopper A.** The older persons' assessment and liaison team 'OPAL': evaluation of comprehensive geriatric assessment in acute medical inpatients. Age Ageing. 2007;**36**(6):670–5.

25 BaztanJJ, Suarez-Garcia FM, Lopez-Arrieta J, et al. Effectiveness of acute geriatric units on functional decline, living at home, and case fatality among older patients admitted to hospital for acute medical disorders: meta-analysis. BMJ. 2009;**338**:b50. doi: 10.1136/bmj.b50

26 Young J, Inouye S. Delirium in older people. BMJ. 2007;**334**: 842–6.

27 Royal College of Physicians. Report of the 2011 inpatient falls pilot audit. London: RCP. Accessed 20 Sep 2013. http://www.rcplondon.ac.uk/sites/default/files/documents/inpatient-falls-final-report-0.pdf

28 Royal College of Psychiatrists. National audit of dementia care in general hospitals 2012–13: second round audit report and update. 2013. Accessed 30 Sep 2013. http://www.rcpsych.ac.uk/pdf/NAD%20NATIONAL%20REPORT%202013.pdf

29 Harari D, Hopper AH, Dhesi J, et al. Proactive Care of Older People undergoing Surgery 'POPS': designing, embedding, evaluating and funding a comprehensive geriatric assessment service for older elective surgical patients. Age Ageing. 2007;**36**:190–6.

30 Devas MB.Geriatric orthopaedics. BMJ. 1974;**1**:190–2.

31 Handoll HHG, Cameron ID, Mak JCS, Finnegan TP. Multidisciplinary rehabilitation for older people with hip fractures. Cochrane Database Syst Rev.2009(4);CD007125. doi: 10.1002/14651858.CD007125.pub2

32 Handoll HHG, Sherrington C, Mak JCS. Interventions for improving mobility after hip fracture surgery in adults. Cochrane Database Syst Rev. 2011(3);CD001704. doi: 10.1002/14651858.CD001704.pub4

33 Vidn M, Serra JA, Moreno C, Riquelme G, Ortiz J. Efficacy of a comprehensive geriatric intervention in older patients hospitalized for hip fracture: a randomized, controlled trial. J Am Geriatr Soc. 2005;**53**(9):1476–82.

34 Marcantonio ER, Flacker JM, Wright RJ, Resnick NM. Reducing delirium after hip fracture: a randomised trial. J Am Geriatr Soc. 2011;**49**(5):516–22.

35 British Orthopaedic Association. The care of patients with fragility fracture. London; BOA; 2007

36 National Hip Fracture Database. Annual report, 2013. Accessed 13 Sep 2013. http://www.nhfd.co.uk/

37 Royal College of Physicians. Medical rehabilitation in 2011 and beyond. Report of a joint working party of the Royal College of Physicians and the British Society of Rehabilitation Medicine. London: RCP; 2010.

38 Covinsky KE, Palmer RM, Fortinsky RH, et al. Loss of independence in activities of daily living in older adults hospitalized with medical illnesses: increased vulnerability with age. J Am Geriatr Soc. 2003;**51**:451–8.

39 Mudge A, O'Rourke P, Denaro CP. Timing and risk factors for functional changes associated with medical hospitalization in older patients. J Gerontol A-Biol. 2010 Aug;**65**(8):866–72.

40 Young Y, Green J, Forster A, et al. Postacute care for older people in community hospitals: A multicenter randomized, controlled trial. J Am Geriatr Soc. 2007;**55**(12):1995–2002.

41 Department of Health. Intermediate care-halfway home. Updated guidance for the NHS and local authorities. London: Department of Health; 2010. Accessed 20 Sep 2013.

http://www.scie-socialcareonline.org.uk/profile.asp?guid=429f6d8f-77aa-45d0-924d-2b1471cb2603

42 **NHS Benchmarking**. National audit of intermediate care report, 2012. http://www.nhsbenchmarking.nhs.uk/icsurvey.aspx

43 **Shepperd S, Doll H, Angus RM, et al**. Admission avoidance hospital at home. Cochrane Database Syst Rev 2008(4);CD007491. doi: 10.1002/14651858.CD007491

44 **Cunliffe AL, Gladman JR, Husbands SL, et al**. Sooner and healthier: a randomised controlled trial and interview study of an early discharge rehabilitation service for older people. Age Ageing. 2004;**33**(3):246–52.

45 **British Geriatrics Society**. Failing the frail: a chaotic approach to commissioning healthcare services for care homes. London: BGS; 2012.

46 **British Geriatrics Society**. A quest for quality in nursing homes. London: BGS; 2011.

47 **Royal College of Physicians**. Improving end-of-life care: professional development for physicians. Report of a working party. London: RCP; 2012. Accessed 27 May 2014. Amber Care Bundle available from http://www.ambercarebundle.org/homepage.aspx

Chapter 5

Therapeutics in older people

Stephen Jackson

Key points

- ◆ Pharmacokinetics in older people is different to that in younger people:
  - renal clearance is lower (water-soluble drugs)
  - hepatic clearance is lower (lipid-soluble drugs)
  - half-life is further prolonged for lipid-soluble drugs because of the increased volume of distribution of such drugs
  - in frail older patients, half-life is further prolonged
    - by reduced hepatic enzyme activity (lipid-soluble drugs)
    - by reduced protein binding and hence increasing the volume of distribution (very heavily protein-bound drugs).
- ◆ Polypharmacy is common and reflects multiple pathology.
- ◆ Inappropriate medication should always be avoided.
- ◆ Methods of enhancing the quality of prescribing include
  - regular medication review
  - prescribing audit using proven indicators of appropriateness
  - education of prescribers.

1 Introduction

The size of the oldest old section of the population is rising and is set to continue to increase (1, Chapter 1). This population has a higher prevalence of chronic illnesses including cardiovascular diseases, cancers, osteoporosis, diabetes, Parkinson's disease, dementia, and many other conditions. An increasing body of research is adding further prescribing indications for diseases that occur in the elderly population. Along with the increasing size of the population, this means that the numbers of prescriptions for elderly patients are increasing. Depending on the age group, between 60% and 80% of elderly people are taking medication and 20% are taking at least five drugs (2). It is also estimated that although those over 75 years account for 14% of the population, they receive 33% of medication prescribed.

2 Age-related changes in physiology and pharmacokinetics

Pharmacokinetics is the description of how the body handles drugs after administration. It incorporates the liberation, absorption, distribution, metabolism, and excretion of drugs and their metabolites. These processes are affected by the physiological changes associated with ageing resulting in changes in the pharmacokinetics of drugs.

2.1 Absorption

Following administration, a number of factors affect a drug's entry into the circulation. These include properties such as particle size, molecular weight, charge, solubility, and pKa (the pH at which 50% remains in a non-ionized, lipid-soluble state). Most drugs are weak acids or bases and are present in solution as both ionized and non-ionized species. Non-ionized drugs are lipid-soluble and diffuse easily across the cell membrane. Following liberation some absorption may take place in the stomach, depending on the pKa of the drug and the pH of the stomach. Gastric acid secretion in response to stimulation decreases with normal ageing. Thus where pH is crucial to ionization, absorption can be affected (e.g. iron compounds). However, for most drugs the large surface area of the small bowel makes it the main site of drug absorption.

With ageing, although many drugs show no change in absorption (3), there is slightly reduced small bowel absorption of some substances (including iron, calcium, and glucose). There is slower colonic transit time with age, and an associated decrease in peristalsis, largely due to a loss of neurons involved in control of the GI tract. Passive intestinal permeability is probably unchanged in old age for most substances. However, active transport of other agents, such as vitamin B12, is impaired. These age-related changes therefore primarily affect drugs with low permeability and low solubility, e.g. cephalexin. Agents such as benzodiazepines (lipid-soluble) and lithium (water-soluble) are readily absorbed.

2.2 Distribution

The volume of distribution (Vd), also known as apparent volume of distribution, is a pharmacological term used to quantify the distribution of a medication between plasma and the rest of the body after oral or parenteral dosing. It is defined as the volume in which an amount of drug would need to be uniformly distributed to produce a given plasma concentration. Put another way, it refers to the fluid volume that would be required to contain the entire drug dose in the body at the same concentration as that in the blood or plasma. A drug with a high Vd (e.g. morphine—300 litres) implies extensive distribution outside the blood or plasma to other tissues such as fat. The Vd is dependent on lipophilicity (increasing the Vd) and the ability of the drug to bind to plasma proteins such as albumin (acidic drugs) and α_1-acid glycoprotein (basic drugs), thus holding the drug in the blood compartment and reducing Vd.

With ageing there is a decrease in lean body weight, muscle mass, and body water, and an increase in body fat per kilogram of body weight. As a result, lipid-soluble drugs such as benzodiazepines, morphine, neuroleptics, and amitriptyline have an increased Vd due to the higher proportion of body fat. With ageing the higher Vd for such lipid-soluble drugs (along with reduced clearance) will result in a prolonged elimination half-life and hence drug effects. For water-soluble drugs, Vd will fall, but clearance will fall to a greater extent.

2.3 **Protein binding**

Many drugs are protein-bound to a varying degree. Bound drugs are inactive. An unbound drug is free to mediate its effect. The binding is usually reversible. Most acidic drugs (e.g. ibuprofen, diazepam, phenytoin, warfarin) bind to albumin. Basic drugs such as lidocaine and tricyclic antidepressants bind to α_1-acid glycoprotein. With healthy ageing there is no substantial change in plasma proteins; however, intercurrent illness can result in a drop in albumin and an increase in $\alpha1$-acid glycoprotein (an acute phase protein). Chronic disease tends to accelerate the age-related decline in serum albumin. This can produce clinically significant increases in the free fraction of very heavily protein-bound drugs such as ibuprofen (99.5% bound). Other highly protein-bound drugs include benzodiazepines (>90%) and many antipsychotics (>90%). In contrast, some drugs are not protein-bound at all (e.g. lithium).

2.4 **Clearance—hepatic**

Hepatic metabolism of drugs is dependent on the ability of the liver to extract drugs from the blood passing through the organ. Lipophilic drugs are metabolized into more hydrophilic compounds that are eliminated mainly through the urine. However, in some cases metabolites are biologically active or even toxic. Thus risperidone is metabolized to an active metabolite (9-OH risperidone), which has an elimination half-life (t1/2z) of 22 hours versus the parent drug t1/2z of 4 hours. Similarly, diazepam is metabolized to an active metabolite (desmethyl diazepam), amitriptyline is metabolized to nortriptyline, and morphine is metabolized to the active metabolite morphine-6-glucuronide. In the liver, phase I metabolism introduces a functional group onto the parent compound, generally resulting in loss of pharmacological activity. Several studies have shown an age-related decline in the clearance of drugs by phase I metabolism, probably reflecting a reduced hepatic mass as enzyme activity is preserved. Induction, or increased synthesis of the cytochrome P450 enzymes induced by drugs such as phenytoin, isoniazid, glucocorticoids, and alcohol, may decrease the bioavailability of parent drug compounds.

Inhibition of drug metabolism enzymes, commonly by depletion of necessary co-factors, results in elevated levels of parent drugs. This can lead to increased pharmacological effects and an increased incidence of drug-induced toxicity. Inhibition of different isoforms of cytochrome P450 enzymes can be seen with erythromycin and ketoconazole (CYP450 3A4) and SSRIs (CYP450 2D6). For two of these enzymes, CYP4502D6 and CYP4502C19, genetic polymorphisms exist that lead to poorly functioning enzymes causing individuals to be poor metabolizers. Thus when prescribing drugs metabolized by these enzymes where the therapeutic window is narrow, prescribing should be on the basis that the patient is a poor metabolizer. For example, when prescribing haloperidol, starting doses should be appropriately low in poor CYP2D6 metabolizers.

2.5 **Clearance—renal**

Excretion of drugs and metabolites in the urine involves three processes: glomerular filtration, active tubular secretion, and passive tubular reabsorption. With ageing, renal mass decreases, as does the glomerular filtration rate (GFR). There is also a reduced ability to concentrate urine and a reduced thirst during water deprivation.

Davies and Shock, in a classic cross-sectional inulin clearance study, demonstrated that GFR decreases by about 8ml/min/1.73 m² per decade from the fourth decade onwards (4). There is wide individual variability in the age-related fall in GFR, further amplified by the presence of vascular and renal disease. Creatinine clearance is influenced by nutritional status, protein intake, muscle mass, body weight, gender, and ethnicity. As people age, muscle mass is reduced and daily urinary creatinine excretion decreases, accompanied by a reduction in creatinine clearance. The combined effect of these changes is that declining GFR in older patients is accompanied by lower rises in serum creatinine than would occur in younger people.

Reduction in GFR with age affects the clearance of many drugs such as water-soluble antibiotics, diuretics, lithium, and water-soluble non-steroidal anti-inflammatory drugs. GFR can be estimated using several equations. The Cockcroft and Gault equation uses age, weight, gender, and serum creatinine (5):

$$\text{GFR (mls/min)} = 1.23 \times (140\text{-age}) \text{ (years)} \times \text{weight (kg)} \times (0.85 \text{ if female})/72 \times \text{Creatinine } (\mu\text{mol/L})$$

The National Service Framework for Kidney Disease recommended that all laboratories report a formula-based estimation of GFR when serum creatinine is requested in adults. The Modification of Diet in Renal Disease (MDRD) study equation (based on serum creatinine, age, gender, and ethnic group) (6) is widely used. The MDRD formula has the advantage of not requiring a weight, and can therefore be issued by the laboratory at the same time as a creatinine result is reported. It takes no direct account of muscle mass. It estimates the reduction in muscle bulk on the basis of the average reduction due to age. The classification of chronic kidney disease (Box 5.1) is based on eGFR estimated by the MDRD formula. The Cockcroft and Gault formula tends to estimate lower values for GFR than MDRD estimates. Some data suggest that the MDRD formula is unreliable in end-stage renal disease (7).

The adjustment of drug dosing in elderly patients becomes particularly relevant where drugs are substantially or entirely excreted by the kidneys. The

Box 5.1   Stages of chronic kidney disease (CKD)

Stage	GFR*	Description	Treatment stage
1	90+	Normal kidney function but urine findings or structural abnormalities or genetic trait point to kidney disease	Observation, control of blood pressure.
2	60–89	Mildly reduced kidney function, and other findings (as for stage 1) point to kidney disease	Observation, control of blood pressure and risk factors.
3A 3B	45–59 30–44	Moderately reduced kidney function	Observation, control of blood pressure and risk factors.
4	15–29	Severely reduced kidney function	Planning for end-stage renal failure.
5	<15 or on dialysis	Very severe, or end-stage kidney failure (sometimes call established renal failure)	Treatment choices.

*All GFR (glomerular filtration rate) values are normalized to an average body surface area (size) of 1.73m^2

Acknowledgement: The Renal Association—original authors Goddard J, Harris K, and Turner N. <http://www.renal.org/information-resources/the-uk-eckd-guide/ckd-stages#sthash.yN5edpAX.orJDyUxb.dpbs>

exception to this rule is where the therapeutic window is wide, such as with penicillin. In this situation dosage modification is not needed, as high concentrations are not associated with an increase in adverse drug reactions. Routine pre-prescribing estimation of GFR is an essential adjunct to good prescribing in this vulnerable group. Given that the MDRD eGFR is now routinely provided, this is the method of choice.

Where there is a narrow therapeutic window, significant toxicity can occur if doses are not adjusted downwards to account for renal impairment and subsequent reduced excretion. Examples include lithium, aminoglycosides, and digoxin.

The presence of causes of chronic kidney disease such as hypertension and diabetes will potentiate the age-associated decline in renal function. It is especially important to review regularly drug therapy in frail older patients who may have, along with other known cardiovascular morbidities, undetected but significant renal dysfunction.

2.6 Elimination half-life

The elimination half-life (t1/2z) is the time it takes for the plasma concentration to be reduced by 50% during the elimination phase. This is distinct from the absorption half-life (t1/2abs) or distribution half-life (t1/2$_1$). It is a function of both volume of distribution and clearance, where clearance is the nominal volume of blood that is cleared of drug per unit time:

$$t1/2z \propto Vd/Cl$$

where t1/2z = elimination half-life; Vd = volume of distribution; Cl = clearance.

The t1/2z provides a good indication of the time required to achieve steady state after a drug is started. It also provides an estimate of the time required to remove a drug from the body, and of appropriate dosing intervals. It takes approximately five half-lives to reach steady state during chronic dosing and a similar time to remove the drug when dosing is stopped. Thus for amiodarone, with a t1/2z in excess of two months during chronic dosing in elderly patients (8), it would take at least ten months to reach steady state or to remove the drug from the body. For lipid-soluble drugs, the elimination half-life increases with age, due to both reduced clearance and increased V (9). For water-soluble drugs such as lithium, the reduced volume of distribution partially offsets the effect of reduced clearance on t1/2z.

Renal tubular interactions are a common cause of pharmacokinetic drug interactions. For example, renal tubular reabsorption of lithium is increased by thiazide and loop diuretics. This leads to reduced clearance of lithium and hence rising concentrations. Thus therapeutic drug monitoring can help manage such interactions, unlike pharmacodynamic interactions when concentrations do not change.

3 Polypharmacy and multiple pathology

One of the hallmarks of an ageing population is the accumulation of multiple diseases where pathology affecting many organ systems within an individual is seen and is referred to as *frailty*, which is associated with its own poor prognosis (Chapter 7). This is in contrast to individuals who have isolated pathology.

Polypharmacy is common in older people, with approximately 20% of people aged over 70 years taking five or more medications (2). From 1996–2006 the average number of items prescribed to people aged 60 and over almost doubled from 21.2 to 40.8 items per person per year (10). Polypharmacy is derived from the Greek, meaning 'many medications', but it has come to mean 'too many medications'. This interpretation is incorrect, however, as all of the prescribed medications may have an appropriate indication.

Polypharmacy is associated with increases in many adverse outcomes, including drug interactions, adverse drug reactions, falls, hospital admissions, length of stay, readmission rate soon after discharge, and mortality rate (11). However, these effects are likely be due to polypharmacy acting as a marker of multiple pathology or frailty, as opposed to being an independent risk factor. A number of medications pose particular risks for elderly patients (Box 5.2).

Box 5.2 Examples of drugs that pose particular risk for older patients

Medication	Adverse Drug Reaction
Long-term use of non-steroidal anti-inflammatory drugs	Gastrointestinal haemorrhage, renal impairment, antagonism of antihypertensive drugs
Benzodiazepines	Falls due to balance impairment
Anticholinergic medications	Unmasking Alzheimer's disease, delirium, urinary retention
Tricyclic antidepressants	Orthostatic hypotension, sedation, dry mouth
Chlorpropamide	Hypoglycaemia
Doxazosin	Orthostatic hypotension, urinary continence problems

4 Inappropriate prescribing

Inappropriate prescribing as a concept has the advantage over the term polypharmacy as it seeks to address both prescribing without rationale or evidence and the absence of prescribing when there is an indication. The latter is particularly important in the context of evidence-based prophylaxis such as heparin prophylaxis of venous thromboembolism, antithrombotic prophylaxis of stroke in atrial fibrillation, and fracture prophylaxis in osteoporosis. Apart from being unnecessary, inappropriate medication contributes to the risk of an adverse drug reaction that is directly related to the number of medications being taken.

5 Atypical presentation and response to medication (pharmacodynamics)

Adjustments in dose, formulation, and delivery need to be made according to the age and frailty of the patient. Some drugs are best avoided altogether, including benzodiazepines, anticholinergic drugs, and long-acting hypoglycaemic agents. Problems arise when older patients are assumed to respond to medications in the same way that younger adults do. A related confounding factor is that an older patient's underlying pathology may present differently. For example, the prevalence of painless peptic ulceration is high, as is painless myocardial infarction.

6 How can inappropriate prescribing in older people be reduced?

6.1 Good prescribing practice

A set of simple rules can go a long way towards maintaining good prescribing practice. Some of these guidelines, such as using as few prescribers as possible, are evidence-based (12), but the majority, due to the paucity of evidence in this area, are consensus opinion (Box 5.3).

6.2 Medication review

The National Service Framework for Older People recommended regular medication reviews, with patients taking more four or more medications being reviewed every six months and those taking fewer reviewed annually (13). General practitioners, who do most of the prescribing, have the facility of setting the authorisation of repeat prescriptions for a period of time or a number of repeats, automatically generating a recall from their clinical software. Medication review for all patients being prescribed four or more repeat medicines is part of the quality and outcomes framework of the GP contract.

Box 5.3 Guidelines for good prescribing in elderly patients

- Carry out a regular medication review and discuss and agree on all changes with the patient.
- Stop any current drugs that are not indicated.
- Prescribe new drugs that have a clear indication.
- If possible, avoid drugs that have known deleterious effects in elderly patients, such as benzodiazepines, or recommend dosage reduction when appropriate.
- Use the recommended dosages for elderly patients.
- Use simple drug regimens and appropriate administration systems.
- Consider using once daily or once weekly formulations and using fixed dose combinations when possible.
- Consider non-pharmacological therapies, if appropriate.
- Limit the number of prescribers per patient, if possible.
- Where possible, avoid treating adverse drug reactions with further medication.

The medication review examines not only the indication and dosage of existing medications but provides an opportunity for the identification and treatment of new conditions such as atrial fibrillation, cardiac failure, and Alzheimer's disease, which increase in prevalence with advancing age. Older people with complex medication or medical needs should be referred for a specialist review by a geriatrician.

A systematic review of the effects of interventions led by pharmacists in reducing polypharmacy identified only 14 trials meeting the inclusion criteria, and these tended to report cost savings rather than benefits to the patients (2). A randomized controlled trial found that regular telephone counselling by a hospital pharmacist increased concordance and reduced all-cause mortality without altering the total number of medications taken (14), but it would be difficult to implement this intervention in the wider community. The 2005 contract for community pharmacists included a medicines use review as the first advanced level service to be implemented, but this is aimed at ensuring medication is taken and taken properly. Without the clinical records, pharmacists cannot review the indications for treatment. Community pharmacists have an important role in spotting adverse drug reactions, interactions, and compliance problems, even though there is no evidence that this reduces mortality or emergency admissions (15).

6.3 Using as few prescribers as possible

In the UK the majority of prescribing is undertaken by a patient's general practitioner, but treatment is often initiated or adjusted in secondary care, so good communication is crucial. Unintentional discrepancies in medication are found in half of older patients after they have left hospital, an error rate that can be halved if the community pharmacist is sent a copy of the discharge summary (16).

A study in the US demonstrated that the incidence of adverse drug reactions is directly related to the number of prescribing physicians (12). The effect of non-medical prescribing is uncertain. It results in a similar number of prescriptions to physician prescribing, but increases the potential number of prescribers, although independent nurse prescribers usually work in close cooperation with a medical prescriber.

6.4 Education

A Cochrane review concluded that educational outreach visits appear to be a promising approach to modifying health professional behaviour, especially prescribing (17). In a UK study of 75 randomly selected general practices, there was a small improvement in prescribing practice in those assigned educational outreach (18). Interestingly, smaller practices (two or fewer full-time equivalent practitioners) improved by 13.5% whereas larger practices did not improve significantly. This may have resulted from the greater attendance of doctors at the outreach meetings. We previously showed that similar interventions in a randomized controlled trial in hospital practice also resulted in changed prescribing versus usual care (19).

6.5 Electronic prescribing

Electronic prescribing aims to reduce prescribing and administration errors by eliminating the risk of errors in generating or reading the traditional paper prescription. This is one step toward the overall goal of integrating the entire patient record across the health service in order to minimize errors and delays in communication between the variety of service providers. Decision support can be integrated within this structure. An early indication of benefit is given by a before-and-after study in a surgical ward of a London teaching hospital. The study showed a reduction in prescribing and medication administration errors, and fewer prescription endorsements by a pharmacist, following the introduction of closed-loop electronic prescribing (20).

6.6 **Audit**

Auditing of prescribing is integral to providing good clinical care, but the problem of the traditional audit loop of data gathering, interpretation, and feedback is that the long delay between an action and its consequent feedback reduces any impact on behaviour. Furthermore, amalgamated data distances the prescriber from specific errors, making it harder to see an obvious way to improve. Audit does not necessarily change behaviour, but prescribing indicators have been developed for older patients (21, 22) which could provide immediate feedback when integrated into electronic prescribing systems.

7 **Future directions**

One of the greatest challenges within the field of drug treatment for elderly patients is the expansion of the evidence base to include the patients who will receive drug treatments. Historically the problem has been the failure to include older patients in clinical trials in a whole range of therapeutic areas. Older patients are often excluded from studies by the trial design. Even when they are included, the prevalence of those with chronic disease and frailty is very low. While there is now some recognition that inclusion and exclusion criteria must change, frail older patients are difficult to recruit and study. This is partly because of reduced ability to take part and partly because such patients and their carers are more likely to refuse to take part than fitter patients. A separate problem is that even when there are data that extend the licensed indication for a drug to include frail older patients, this rarely results in the extension of the marketing authorization. This results in off-label prescribing even when there is an evidence base.

Much is known about age-related and disease-related changes in pharmacokinetics but implementation of this knowledge is suboptimal. While specialists in geriatric medicine have received training in the areas addressed by this chapter, a vast amount of prescribing is undertaken in primary care and other hospital specialties where such skills are not as well developed. There is thus a challenge relating to education and training. The slow implementation of prescribing indicators as a way of documenting the quality of prescribing is an important step towards improvement.

8 **Conclusion**

A number of well-recognized changes in the pharmacokinetics of drugs are associated with ageing which have important implications for prescribing. Most notable is the prolongation of elimination half-life and the consequent need for lower daily doses. The multiple medications often taken by older patients need regular review but are not necessarily to be avoided. Methods of enhancing the quality of prescribing, such as medication review, prescribing audit, and education are to be encouraged as they also reflect good prescribing practice.

Websites relevant to this chapter

National Service Framework for Older People—sets out the government's quality standards for health and social care services for older people.

<https://www.gov.uk/government/publications/quality-standards-for-care-services-for-older-people>

Medicines and older people implementing medicines-related aspects of the NSF for older people.

<http://webarchive.nationalarchives.gov.uk/+/www.dh.gov.uk/en/publicationsandstatistics/publications/publicationspolicyandguidance/DH_4,008,020>

Centre for Pharmacy Postgraduate Education (CPPE) is a useful resource on common presentations in elderly patients and their treatment.

<http://www.cppe.ac.uk/learning/Details.asp?TemplateID=Older-D-02&Format=D&ID=0&EventID=39,396>

National Service Framework for Kidney Disease—sets out the government's quality standards for kidney disease care.

<https://www.gov.uk/government/publications/national-service-framework-kidney-disease>

References

1 **Office for National Statistics**. Mid-year population estimates. ONS; 2010. http://www.statistics.gov.uk/cci/nugget.asp?id=949

2 **Rollason V, Vogt N**. Reduction of polypharmacy in the elderly: a systematic review of the role of the pharmacist. Drugs Aging. 2003;**20**:817–32.

3 **Gainsborough N, Maskrey VL, Nelson ML, Keating J, Sherwood RA, Jackson SHD, Swift CG**. The association of age with gastric emptying. Age Ageing. 1993;**22**:37–40.

4 **Davies DF, Shock NW**. Age changes in glomerular filtration rate, effective renal plasma flow, and tubular excretory capacity in adult males. J Clin Invest. 1950;**29**:496–507.

5 **Cockcroft DW, Gault MH**. Prediction of creatinine clearance from serum creatinine. Nephron. 1976;**16**:31–41.

6 **Levey AS, Bosch JP, Lewis JB, Greene T, Rogers N, Roth D**; Modification of Diet in Renal Disease Study Group. A more accurate method to estimate glomerular filtration rate from serum creatinine: a new prediction equation. Ann Intern Med. 1999;**130**:461–70.

7 Grootendorst DC, Michels WM, Richardson JD, Jager KJ, Boeschoten EW, Dekker FW, Krediet RT; NECOSAD Study Group. The MDRD formula does not reflect GFR in ESRD patients. Nephrol Dial Transplant. 2011;**26**:1932–7.

8 Latini R, Tognoni G, Kates RE. Clinical pharmacokinetics of amiodarone. Clin Pharmacokinet. 1984;**9**:136–56.

9 Zeeh J, Platt D. The aging liver: structural and functional changes and their consequences for drug treatment in old age. Clin Pharmacol Ther. 2002;**71**:115–21.

10 Health Survey for England, 2007. www.hscic.gov.uk/pubs/hse07healthylifestyles

11 Frazier SC. Health outcomes and polypharmacy in elderly individuals. J Gerontol Nurs 2005;**31**:4–11.

12 Green JL, Hawley JN, Rask KJ. Is the number of prescribing physicians an independent risk factor for adverse drug events in an elderly outpatient population? Am J Geriatr Pharmacother. 2007;5:31–9.

13 Department of Health. Medicines and older people: implementing medicines-related aspects of the NSF for older people. 2001. http://www.dh.gov.uk/prod_consum_dh/groups/dh_digitalassets/@dh/@en/documents/digitalasset/dh_4067247.pdf

14 Wu JYF, Leung WYS, Chang, S et al. Effectiveness of telephone counselling by a pharmacist in reducing mortality in patients receiving polypharmacy: randomised controlled trial. BMJ. 2006;**333**:522–7.

15 Bond C, Matheson C, Williams S, Williams P, Donnan P. Repeat prescribing: a role for community pharmacists in controlling and monitoring repeat prescriptions. Brit J Gen Pract. 2000;**50**:271–5.

16 Duggan C, Feldman R, Hough J, Bates I. Reducing adverse prescribing discrepancies following hospital discharge. Int J Pharm Pract 1998;**6**:77–82.

17 O'Brien T, Oxman AD, Davis DA, Haynes RB, Freemantle N, Harvey EL. Educational outreach visits: effects on professional practice and health care outcomes. Cochrane Database Syst Rev. 2000;2:CD000409.

18 Freemantle N, Nazareth I, Eccles M, Wood J, Haines A. Evidence-based OutReach trialists. A randomised controlled trial of the effect of educational outreach by community pharmacists on prescribing in UK general practice. Br J Gen Pract. 2002;**52**:290–5.

19 Batty GM, Oborne CA, Hooper R, Jackson SHD. Investigating intervention strategies to increase the appropriate use of benzodiazepines in elderly medical in-patients. Brit J Clin Governance. 2001;**6**: 252–8.

20 Franklin BD, O'Grady K, Donyai P, Jacklin A, Barber N. The impact of a closed-loop electronic prescribing and administration system on prescribing errors, administration errors and staff time: a before-and-after study. Qual Saf Health Care. 2007;**16**:279–84.

21 Oborne CA, Batty GM, Maskrey V, Swift CG, Jackson SHD. Development of prescribing indicators for elderly medical patients. Brit J Clin Pharmacol. 1997;**43**: 91–7.

22 Gallagher PF, O'Connor MN, O'Mahony D. Prevention of potentially inappropriate prescribing for elderly patients: a randomized controlled trial using STOPP/START criteria. Clin Pharmacol Ther. 2011;**89**:845–54.

Chapter 6

Dementia and memory clinics

Alistair Burns, Richard Atkinson, Sean Page, and David Jolley

Key points

- Memory clinics provide a valuable service for the assessment and management of people with memory difficulties.
- They have also provided a focus for the initiation and monitoring of antidementia drug treatments.
- They have grown in number and range of services they provide over the years.
- A robust accreditation programme exists to assess the services and service standards.
- As the number of people coming forward for investigation of memory problems increases, memory clinics may need realigning more to community and primary care settings.

1 Introduction

The ideas of health in later life that were developed by forward-thinking physicians in the nineteenth century such as Cheyne (1724) and Day (1849), cited by Grimley Evans (1), grew to what we know of today as geriatric medicine. Through pioneering efforts within the UK in the early twentieth century the speciality was nurtured within the ever-evolving structure of the NHS (Chapter 1). Mental health services in the UK of the 1940s and 1950s were based in mental hospitals. With few exceptions, such as Felix Post, a psychiatrist working at the Maudsley Hospital in London, psychiatrists were not interested in older people or the disorders which affected them. However, they complained that mental hospitals were becoming congested and threatened to be overwhelmed by the number of people with 'senile dementia' that presented in advanced stages from the growing population who were aged 65 years and above. Thus it was that pioneers of geriatric medicine took on with interest the mental disorders they encountered among their patients in wards and in the community, seeking help from psychiatry only when matters (usually behavioural problems) became extreme. This process of British physicians building on research concepts to deliver health services has been replicated numerous times, notably in the development of service-oriented memory clinics.

The first British memory clinic, inspired by examples from the USA, was established at the Geriatric Research Unit at University College London in 1983 (2). More clinics followed at the Maudsley Hospital (3) and Cardiff (4, 5). These were research ventures involving psychologists, geriatricians, psychiatrists, and sometimes other staff. They began to see patients who had not previously come to specialist services and whose memory problems were usually mild to moderate and potentially responsive to interventions. This experience contrasted with reports that dementia care at the time often consisted of erratic, ad hoc response to individuals and families and other care agencies at times of crisis (6).

There are approximately 800,000 people currently living with dementia in the UK. Over the next 30 years this number has been confidently predicted to double (7). Recent research suggests that improved general health and the reduction of vascular risk factors from middle age onwards, together with the prescription of thrombolytic and lipid-lowering medicines, are reducing the incidence and prevalence of dementia (8). This is good news, but the numbers still remain high. There has been recognition for at least 50 years that dementia is often not identified or diagnosed (9). The Alzheimer's Society, using national data, concluded that only 46% of people with dementia in the UK had received a formal diagnosis (<www.alzheimers.org.uk/dementiamap>). It seems that the stigma about dementia is having significant negative effects on the diagnosis and management of dementia. The worry is that people are missing out on potentially useful treatments and help. Not having problems recognized and being short-changed by services leads to great frustration and distress; better practices must be identified, resourced, and provided.

2 Development of memory clinics

Memory clinics have been developed with the aim of improving the diagnosis of dementia and thereby improving the care and support that people with dementia and their families receive. When memory clinics were established in the 1980s, they had a number of objectives (Box 6.1) and tended to concentrate expertise within specialist centres, usually within hospitals. Although clearly an area of particular interest to old-age psychiatrists, the development of hospital memory clinics along these lines was almost counter to the genesis of old-age psychiatry, which had had a transformative effect on mental health services for older people and aimed to take services into the community (10). Clinics were, and still are, often associated with university departments and led by physicians or neurologists, though increasingly psychiatrists and psychologists are lead clinicians (11, 12).

Box 6.1 Objectives of the first memory clinics

- to forestall deterioration in dementia by early diagnosis and treatment
- to identify and treat disorders other than dementia that might be contributing to the patient's problems
- to evaluate new therapeutic agents in the treatment of dementia
- to reassure people who are worried that they might be losing their memory, when no morbid deficits are found.

Memory clinics' original guiding principles are still recognized. The Information Centre definition of 2011 states that memory clinics should 'aid the early detection and diagnosis of dementia' and 'provide early intervention to maximise quality of life and independent functioning and to manage risk and prevent future harm to older people with memory difficulties and their carers' (13).

Memory services within the NHS have proved popular. A survey in 1993 identified 20 throughout the UK and Ireland (14). This figure rose to 102 in 2002. This rise may partly have been due to the licensing of anticholinesterase drugs for the treatment of dementia (15) and the recommendation by the National Institute of Clinical Excellence (NICE) that cholinesterase inhibitors should be prescribed, by specialists, and only for people with mild to moderate Alzheimer's disease (16).

Further encouragement came from the Department of Health when, in 2009, Primary Care Trust funding for dementia services was increased. By 2011 there were 337 commissioned memory services in England alone with plans for a further 106 services to be rolled out in the following year (13).

Most of the newer clinics and memory services have been created in districts which are not centres of excellence for research. In the UK (15), most are linked to mental health services, usually within the department for psychiatry in later life, though some clinics are led by physicians or neurologists (10, 12). Scrutiny to determine the best value of memory services (17, 18), together with notes of caution (19) and review of actual practice (20), have begun to refine understanding of their worth.

Approaches to defining and improving standards have begun internationally (21). In the UK, the Royal College of Psychiatrists (Box 6.2) provides an accreditation service that uses criteria agreed in consensus on aspects of structure and function to monitor services and encourage provision of best practice (22). This has allowed the creation of a register of accredited services and this is being used to facilitate audits that inform comparisons between services and rolling programmes for improvement.

Box 6.2 Memory services' accreditation from the Royal College of Psychiatrists

- ◆ The Royal College of Psychiatrists sought to address the lack of uniformity by introducing the Memory Services National Accreditation Programme (MSNAP) in 2009.
- ◆ A series of Internet links are available which share the work and benefits of this service:
  - <www.rcpsych.ac.uk/workinpsychiatry/qualityimprovement/ qualityandaccreditation/memoryservices/memory servicesaccreditation.aspx>
  - <www.rcpsych.ac.uk/workinpsychiatry/qualityimprovement/ qualityandaccreditation/memoryservices/memoryservices accreditation/memoryservicesforum2013.aspx>
  - <www.rcpsych.ac.uk/pdf/Hodge%20Sophie.pdf>
  - <http://www.rcpsych.ac.uk/PDF/MSNAP%20National%20Report% 202011-12.pdf>

---

3 What are the characteristics of a memory clinic?

Previous reviews have asked: what do memory clinics do, and what do they achieve? (11, 12).

3.1 What do they do?

Memory clinics are multifunctional and provide various services (Box 6.3).

They bring together a team: doctors, psychologists, nurses, occupational therapists, sometimes social workers, speech and language therapists, dieticians, clinical pharmacologists, and others. Voluntary organizations may contribute support and encourage links that will be useful for the future.

Box 6.3 What memory clinics do

- team formation
- infrastructure
- assessment clinics
- treatment and rehabilitation
- social interventions and support for carers
- advice on benefits and legal issues
- liaison with other agencies
- education and training
- health promotion
- follow-up to end of life
- research and audit.

They provide a place: and particular time slots where people come together. People in the team learn from each other and are available to patients and carers and there is a venue where patients and carers meet and know they are not on their own.

Clinics provide assessment: medical, psychological and functional, social, benefits, legal, and spiritual. A provisional diagnosis and formulation with an initial plan of action should be available from the first contact. This may include the need for additional investigations or simply to wait to see what time will bring. It can be shared with the GP, patient, and carers, and with other agencies with the agreement of the patient (22, 23).

Treatment and rehabilitation: possibilities span medical interventions; psychological interventions; other therapies, including pets, music, art, exercise, and 'alternative therapies' such as massage and multisensory stimulation (24).

Social interventions and support for carers: include counselling and explanations where indicated as well as help in negotiating additional support to complement what families and friends are pleased and able to contribute.

Advice on benefits and legal issues: including safety at home and when driving.

Liaison with other agencies: often with social services, the independent sector, and care homes.

Education and training: may focus on staff of the clinic and the people who come as students, trainees, and visitors. It includes patients and informal carers. Clinics are increasingly drawn to activities that raise awareness of dementia and similar conditions in the wider community, and especially to improve the competence and confidence of professionals in other caring organizations such as care homes, hospitals, and support services in their dealings with people with dementia.

Health promotion: follows naturally from educational initiatives. There is encouraging evidence that approaches to improved general health are responsible for a fall in incidence and prevalence of dementia while survival with dementia is prolonged as a consequence of better-informed life with the condition (10).

Follow-up to end of life: what is to be done in the long life which many people with dementia and similar conditions will live is crucial to the worth of clinics. The numbers determine that not everyone with dementia can or need be involved with a specialist clinic throughout the course of this altered life. It is, however, essential that there is a system in place which guarantees competent, flexible, and responsive support through to death and support of families beyond this. Integration of activities, involving clinics but especially primary care and sometimes a hospice, is a pattern which is becoming realized (25, 26).

Research and audit: memory clinics began as research centres and specialist clinics; they continue to lead the field in research of all kinds.

The multidisciplinary nature of memory clinics encourages collaboration between geriatricians, psychogeriatricians, and psychologists. This collaboration has led to a wealth of interesting and innovative research projects that have helped to advance our knowledge and understanding of the processes involved in dementia syndromes. Notable research from these groups, such as Peter Crome's memory clinic in Stoke-on-Trent, has considered the role of cholinesterase inhibitors (27) and enabled the 'aluminium theory' of Alzheimer's disease to be investigated (28).

The work of the South Manchester clinic exemplifies the continued evolution of the memory clinic model. Inspired by pioneers including Raymond Levy (3), the multidisciplinary team have modified and evaluated the roles of team members, including the role of nurse specialists and the concept of distributed responsibility, as well as utilizing opportunities for research (29, 30).

3.2 **What do they achieve?**

Clinics encourage people to come forward more readily and at times of less impairment than was the case when the only option was routine geriatric or psychogeriatric care. However, some people find attendance at any type of clinic daunting and others simply will not attend (31). Memory clinics have reduced the stigma associated with labels such as 'mental' or 'geriatric', although there remains a challenge in reaching people from ethnic minority groups (31). Assessment, investigation, diagnosis, and communication of these are generally appreciated (32). Many people are lacking in knowledge about the conditions which cause memory problems and which may progress as dementia. They and their families can benefit from teaching sessions in groups and individually (33, 34).

4 **The future of memory clinics**

The number of people with dementia and related disorders and of people quite properly concerned about altered memory is growing. The demand for memory services has increased beyond the capabilities of memory clinics as originally conceived. The search for alternative models includes closer collaboration between specialist and primary care, and drives to increase competence and confidence in identifying and supporting people with dementia and similar disorders within and by all components of a caring community.

The aim is to break down barriers to access to initial assessment and diagnosis. This might be done by increasing the capacity and changing the mode of operation of clinics (35). An alternative is for clinic staff to give part of their week to work in primary care in the familiar setting of a person's local GP surgery (26, 36). These innovations seek to reduce stigma and simplify logistical problems when people seek help for memory problems.

5 **Conclusion**

- Memory clinics have transformed the way in which people with memory problems have been assessed and appropriately managed.
- They have successfully adapted over the years from specialist settings to being integral to community-based services.
- They offer a focus for service excellence, dissemination of good practice, and opportunities for research and audit.
- The UK has led the field in the development of memory clinics and setting standards.
- New models of memory clinics that are community based and link with primary care need to be developed and evaluated.

Services in the UK for older people with mental health problems, including dementia, have been transformed since the introduction of comprehensive specialist community-oriented psychogeriatric services from the late 1960s onwards. These services drew strength and inspiration from geriatric medicine and the two specialties have continued to learn together. The introduction of memory clinics in the 1980s, transplanted from the USA and pioneered by geriatricians but welcomed by psychiatrists and neurologists, has helped to increase the acceptability, quality, and breadth of services for people with dementia and related disorders. They also provide a setting where research and audit can be most easily conducted. In addition, they offer an identifiable reference point for professionals and lay people interested in and involved in care of people with dementia.

Their adoption by so many countries internationally is a demonstration of the recognition of their worth and potential in providing services such as education, awareness, and training as well as a platform for research and audit. Questions relating to the best way of applying knowledge of their strengths and limitations and alternative configurations demonstrate healthy open-mindedness within the community of clinicians, researchers, and others who devote their lives to this work.

Acknowledgement

Many thanks to Susan Jolley for reading the manuscript and contributing ideas and comments.

Websites and key guidelines relevant to this chapter

An update on the prime minister's dementia challenge:

<http://dementiachallenge.dh.gov.uk/>

Royal College of General Practitioners on dementia:

<http://www.rcgp.org.uk/clinical-and-research/clinical-resources/dementia.aspx>

Advice on what cognitive tests to use:

<http://www.alzheimers.org.uk/cognitiveassessment>

Resources to support the dementia prevalence calculator

<http://www.dementiapartnerships.org.uk/diagnosis>

Information about memory services:

<http://www.rcpsych.ac.uk/workinpsychiatry/qualityimprovement/qualityandaccreditation/memoryservices/memoryservicesaccreditation.aspx>

The range of diagnostic rates across the UK:

<http://www.alzheimers.org.uk/dementiamap>

References

1 Grimley Evans J. Geriatric medicine: a brief history. BMJ. 1997;**315**(7115):1075–7.

2 Van der Cammen T, Simpson J, Fraser R, Preker A, Exton-Smith A. The memory clinic: a new approach to the detection of dementia. Br J Psychiat. 1987;**150**:359–64.

3 Philpot M, Levy R. A memory clinic for the early diagnosis of dementia. Int J Geriatr Psychiat. 1987;**2**:195–200.

4 Bayer A, Richards V, Phillips G. The community memory project: a multi-disciplinary approach to patients with forgetfulness and early dementia. Care of the Elderly. 1990;**2**:236–8.

5 Bayer A, Pathy M, Twining C. The memory clinic. A new approach to the detection of early dementia. Drugs. 1987;**33**(2):84–9.

6 Report of the Royal College of Physicians on organic mental impairment in the elderly. J Roy Coll Phys. 1981;**15**:4–29.

7 Knapp M, Prince M, Albanese E, et al. Dementia UK: the full report. London: Alzheimer's Society; 2007.

8 Matthews F, Arthur A, Barnes LE, et al. A two-decade comparison of prevalence of dementia in individuals aged 65 years and older from three geographical areas of England. Lancet. 2013;**382**(9902):1405–12. doi: 10.1016/S0140-6736(13)61570-6

9 Williamson J, Stokoe IH, Gray S, et al. Old people at home their unreported needs. Lancet. 1964;**i**:117–20.

10 Arie T. The first year of the Goodmayes Psychiatric Service for Old People. Lancet. 1970;**ii**:1179–82.

11 Jolley D, Benbow S, Grizzell M. Memory clinics. Postgrad Med J. 2006;**82**:199–206.

12 Jolley D, Moniz-Cook E. Memory clinics in context. Indian J Psychiat. 2009;**51**:S70–S769.

13 The NHS Information Centre, Community and Mental Health Team. Establishment of memory services—results of a survey of primary care trusts, final figures, 2011. www. hscic.gov.uk/pubs/memoryservicesfinalresults11

14 Wright N, Lindesay J. A survey of memory clinics in the British Isles. Int J Geriatr Psychiat. 1995;**10**(5):379–85.

15 Lindesay J, Marudkar M, van Diepen E, Wilcock G. The second Leicester survey of memory clinics in the British Isles. Int J Geriatr Psychiat. 2002;**17**(1):41–7.

16 National Institute for Clinical Excellence. Guidance on the use of donepezil, rivastigmine and galantamine for the treatment of Alzheimer's disease. Technology Appraisal Guidance No. 19. London: Department of Health; 2001.

17 Iliffe S, Manthorpe J. Evaluating memory clinics. J Roy Soc Med. 2010;**103**(3):81.

18 Iliffe S. Commissioning services for people with dementia. Psychiatrist. 2013;**37**:121–3

19 Le Couteur D, Doust J, Creasey H, Brayne C. Political drive to screen for pre-dementia: not evidence-based and ignores the harms of diagnosis. BMJ. 2013;**347**:f5125. doi: 10.1136/bmj.f5215

20 Foy J. A survey of memory clinic practice in Scotland. Psychiat Bull. 2008;**32**:467–9.

21 Draskovic I, Vernooij-Dassen M, Verhey M, Scheltens P, Rikkert M. Development of quality markers for memory clinics. Int J Geriatr Psychiat. 2008;**23**(2):119–28.

22 Doncaster E, McGeorge M, Orrell M. Developing and implementing quality standards for memory services: The Memory Services National Accreditation Programme (MSNAP). Aging Ment Health. 2011;**15**(1):23–33. doi: 10.1080/13607863.2010.519322

23 Clark M, Benbow S, Scott V, Moreland N, Jolley D. Copying letters to older people in mental health services—policy with unfulfilled potential. Qual Ageing. 2008;**9**(3):31–8.

24 Moniz-Cook E, Manthorpe J. Early psycho-social interventions in dementia: evidence-based practice. London: Jessica Kingsley; 2009.

25 Clark M, Moreland N, et al. Putting personalisation and integration into practice in primary care. J Integrated Care. 2013;**21**(2):105–20.

26 Howard R, McShane R, Lindesay J, Ritchie C, Baldwin A, Barber R, et al. Donepezil and memantine for moderate-to-severe Alzheimer's disease. N Engl J Med. 2012;**366**(10):893–903.

27 Exley C, Korchazhkina O, Job D, Strekopytov S, Polwart A, Crome P. Non-invasive therapy to reduce the body burden of aluminium in Alzheimer's disease. J Alzheimer's Dis. 2006;**10**(1):17–24; discussion 29–31.

28 Page S, Hope K, Bee P, Burns A. Nurses making a diagnosis of dementia—a potential change in practice? Int J Geriatr Psychiat. 2008;**23**(1):27–33.

29 Page S, Hope K, Maj C, Mathew J, Bee P. 'Doing things differently'—working towards distributed responsibility within memory assessment services. Int J Geriatr Psychiat. 2012;**27**(3):280–5.

30 Cooper C, Tandy AR, Balamurali TBS, Livingston G. A systematic review and meta-analysis of ethnic differences in the use of dementia treatment, care, and research. Am J Geriat Psychiat. 2010;**18**(3):193–203.

31 Moniz-Cook E, Woods B. The role of memory clinics and psychosocial interventions in the early stages of dementia. Int J Geriatr Psychiat. 1997;**12**:1143–5.

32 Manthorpe J, Samsi K, Campbell S, et al. From forgetfulness to dementia: commissioning implications of diagnostic experiences. Brit J Gen Pract. 2013;**63**:69–75.

33 Graham C, Ballard C, Sham P. Carers' knowledge of dementia and their expressed concerns. Int J Geriatr Psychiat. 1997;**12**:470–3.

34 Banerjee S, Willis R, Matthews D, Contell F, Chan J, Murray J. Improving the quality of care for mild to moderate dementia: an evaluation of the Croydon Memory Service Model. Int J Geriatr Psychiat. 2007;**22**:782–8.

35 Greening L, Greaves I, Greaves N, Jolley D. Positive thinking on dementia in primary care: Gnosall Memory Clinic. Commun Pract. 2009;**82**(5):20–3.

36 Gnosall Medical Practice. Memory service: the basics. 2012. Accessed 8 Nov 2013. www.gnosallsurgery.co.uk/clinics-and-services.aspx?t=1

37 Jolley D, Greaves I, Clark M. Memory clinics and primary care: not a question of either/or. BMJ. 2012;**344**:e4286.

Chapter 7

Frailty: challenges and progress

Peter Crome and Frank Lally

Key points

- Frailty in older people is characterized by deteriorating health and increasing need for support.
- Frailty has the features of a 'geriatric giant' as originally defined by Isaacs.
- The identification of frail older people is important for medical intervention and for strategic planning.
- The clinical definition of frailty is still being debated but may include the following aspects:
  - a distinct phenotypical profile
  - a frailty index defined by the accumulation of deficits
  - genetic and biochemical predisposition.
- There is no specific treatment for frailty but there are treatments for the diseases that contribute to it.

---

1 Introduction

Frailty, in the context of older people, is a relatively new word to be included in the medical lexicon. The word is derived from the Latin *fragilis* and defined by the dictionary as 'easily broken or destroyed', 'in poor health; weak', and 'morally weak, easily tempted' (1). Despite these rather derogatory and demeaning definitions it has been accepted by the medical community as a way of identifying mainly older people at risk of further decline although the word itself and its concept has its critics (2). A potential pathway to frailty with trigger factors is depicted in Figure 7.1 which is essentially a synopsis of the literature on frailty.

The heterogeneity in health status in older people has been recognized since biblical times. The desirability to define different groups of older people has come more recently from different directions. Within the health community these have arisen from the desire to identify groups of older people who are most at risk of

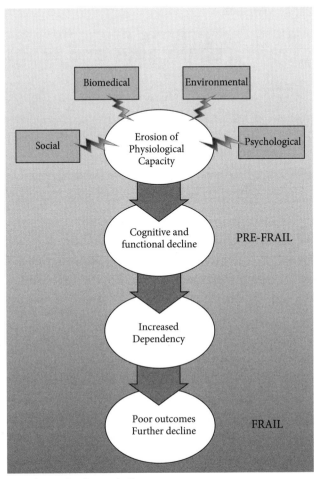

Fig. 7.1 Potential steps leading to frailty.

Factors (boxes) acting either alone or synergistically to reduce physiological capacity leading to increased dependency. This may initially lead to a pre-frail state before tipping into the frailty syndrome leading to further functional decline.

deteriorating health or function. The potential advantages of identifying such people are to allow therapeutic interventions at an individual level and to help plan health and social care services at a population level. Nevertheless, how to define frailty and how best to identify frail individuals has not been resolved.

2 **Definitions**

One of the earliest attempts to define the difference between fit and frail was that of Woodhouse et al. (3). The essential components of the frail person they described were that such people were older, dependent on others for activities of daily living, and often in institutional care. They may not have overt disease but minor abnormalities detected by investigations, and they may be on regular medication. Among the diseases associated with frailty were neurodegenerative conditions (Alzheimer's, Parkinsonism), and arthritis, fractures, and osteoporosis. Both the distinction and the overlap between frailty and chronic diseases continue to be debated (4). Woodhouse and colleagues also drew attention to the physiological changes in later life and the implications for drug therapy. The development of analytical techniques to measure drug pharmacokinetics has allowed major differences to be identified between young and old people. However, it became clear that these differences, which were identified by studying younger volunteers and older hospital patients, were not due to age alone but also to other factors which would now be subsumed into the frailty paradigm. The connection between frailty and prescribing has been a continuing theme of the frailty debate (5).

2.1 **Phenotypes and deficits**

A standard definition of frailty has yet to emerge but two distinct approaches have been suggested: the phenotype and the frailty index. These are in addition to the global clinical impression, which itself may be refined by tools such as the Canadian Study of Health and Aging Frailty Score (6). A recent Delphi consensus approach failed to reach agreement on a specific set of clinical or laboratory biomarkers, although there was agreement on the value of screening for frailty. Consensus was also obtained that the domains of physical performance (including gait speed and mobility), nutritional status, mental health, and cognition should form part of any definition (7).

Fried et al. were the first to establish a frailty phenotype (8) based on a standardized assessment of physical health and has recently been described as rule based (9). Fried defined frailty as comprising three or more of the following characteristics:

+ unintentional weight loss
+ self-reported exhaustion
+ weak grip strength
+ slow walking speed
+ low physical activity.

Using data from the Cardiovascular Health Study of more than 5,000 participants, they found that the presence of frailty for over three years predicted falls, worsening mobility, first hospitalization, and death, with hazard ratios

Table 7.1 The Fried criteria of frailty

Feature	Measurement
Shrinking (sarcopenia)	Unintentional weight loss (>4.5 kg)
Weakness	Lowest quintile of grip strength
Exhaustion	Self-reported using Center of Epidemiological Studies—depression scale
Slow walking speed	Lowest quintile over 15 feet
Low physical activity	kcal/week in lowest quintile

of 2.06, 2.68, 2.25, and 6.47, respectively. People with only one or two of the phenotype factors were at lower risk of adverse outcomes. Fried also drew attention to the difference between frailty (as defined by the phenotype), co-morbidity (presence of many medical conditions), and disability (lack of independence). Subsequently the predictive validity of the phenotype was confirmed by Fried and colleagues using data from the Women's Health and Aging Study (10). The criteria are shown in Table 7.1.

While Fried's methods of identifying frailty may be suitable for epidemiological studies, they are not really practical in the acutely ill or for individuals with severe disability. Additionally they do not take account of psychological, emotional, or cognitive factors that have been shown to have negative health impacts. Simpler criteria have been proposed such as those of Ensrud et al. (11) in which three factors are measured: weight loss of more than 5% between tests, self-reported exhaustion using the Geriatric Depression Scale, and inability to get out of a chair five times without using the arm. However, the latter test may present difficulties for many older people and the height of the chair would be a factor. Montesanto et al. suggested that different populations, such as the older people they studied in Calabria, may represent a unique group with different phenotypical domains identifying frailty (12). Their model employed cognitive functioning, functional activity, physical performance, degree of depression, and self-reported health.

An alternative to the phenotype approach is the frailty index, defined by the accumulation of deficits, which can be physical or mental health diseases, disabilities, or abnormal laboratory findings (13). The more of these deficits a person has, the greater the risk of being frail. A number of such frailty indices have been suggested. Searle et al. (14) proposed a set of criteria that need to be present in constructing a frailty index. According to the authors the criteria must

- be health-related (e.g. not age-related baldness)
- in general increase in prevalence with age
- not become ubiquitous at too early an age (e.g. presbyopia)
- be broad, covering a number of body systems.

They also described a validating process including the determination of cut-off scores based on data from the Yale Precipitating Events Project. Both binary and continuous variables were included. Examples of deficits included are help with bathing, feeling happy, heart attack, and low mini mental state examination. Examples of deficits excluded because they did not meet the Searle et al. (14) criteria are being admitted to hospital in the past year (not age-related) and measured vision. Two European studies that employed a 40-item frailty index confirmed the predictive value of this approach (15, 16). They found that men have a higher mortality rate than women despite having a lower frailty index (15). It has also been suggested that higher physiological functioning in youth may be at the expense of greater susceptibility in later life (17).

The influence of excluding people with disability and subdividing a frailty index into physical health, mental health, and social frailty phenotypes was explored in a study of community-dwelling people over 75 (18). The four-year hazard ratio for death was 3.09 and 2.69 for the physical social types, respectively. The social phenotype, however, did not predict mortality. The frailty index has also been suggested as a way of determining frailty in mouse models (19).

Of course, it must be stated that the presence or absence of frailty is not the only marker of reduced life expectancy or deteriorating function. The presence of advanced cancer is an obvious example of a marker unrelated to frailty.

3 **Frailty and the immune system**

Discussion of the pathophysiological factors reported to be associated with frailty would require a book in its own right. For this reason the authors aim to provide an overview of the burgeoning literature that covers frailty-related immunological and inflammatory predictors with some key references.

Figure 7.2 illustrates some of the potential immunological pathways that may lead to frailty. The illustration is a synopsis of the literature on the subject and gives some of the main factors that have been reported and in which there is still active research interest.

It has been recognized for a long time that as the body ages there are associated biological changes. The term coined for age-related changes to the immune system is immunosenescence. Immunosenescence affects both the innate and

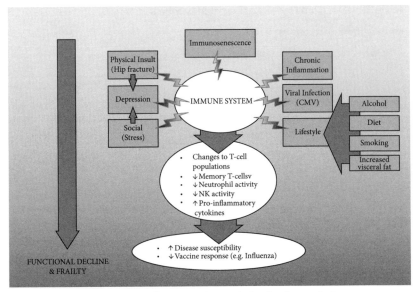

Fig. 7.2 Possible mechanisms of immune dysregulation leading to frailty.

adaptive arms of the immune system. This can lead to changes to white cell populations such as neutrophils and natural killer (NK) cells (innate), as well as to T-lymphocyte subsets (adaptive) such as T-memory cells that allow rapid response to specific antigens already recognized by the system. Other factors can also modify the immune system, such as physical insult and stress. It is recognized that both conditions can lead to depression, which itself is an immune modulator.

The effects of lifestyle choices on our bodies are now well known; factors such as poor diet, excess alcohol, and increased visceral fat have all been implicated. These can cause fluctuations in the levels of circulating cytokines leading to imbalance and/or increased oxidative stress by the production of free radicals, which can have effects on cellular processes and DNA regulation and may lead to cell death (apoptosis).

Chronic inflammation in older people (inflammaging) can also cause a rise in circulating pro-inflammatory cytokines such as tumour necrosis factor alpha (TNF-α) and interleukin 1 (IL-1). C-reactive protein, a marker of inflammation, is often raised in frail or pre-frail individuals.

Many researchers have suggested that a viral infection earlier in life can predispose an individual to immune dysregulation later in life. One often-cited candidate is cytomegalovirus (CMV). This is a common herpes virus and causes little harm at the time of infection. However, it remains within cells and the immune response to it appears to remain raised, thereby placing a burden on the immune system. CMV has been directly associated with frailty in several studies (20, 21).

The upshot is that some or all of these factors can play a part in compromising or regulating the immune system. Lowering responses in the innate arm of the system can lead to increased risk of infections, as cells such as neutrophils and NK cells are not working as they should. Similarly, the immunocompromised individual is unable to produce an adequate response to vaccines such as the influenza vaccine often given to older people during winter months. This adds not only to the physiological burden but also has service and financial implications.

For further reading, some general references on frailty and inflammation are (22–24) and immunosenescence (25–27).

4 **Prevalence**

The prevalence of frailty depends on the population studied and the tool that is used. Fried et al. found an overall prevalence of 7% in people over the age of 65 (8). (Figures in this section have been rounded for clarity.) A systematic review in 2012 showed a range of 4–59% with a weighted average of 10% for frailty and 44% for pre-frailty in 21 studies of community-dwelling over-65s. Not surprisingly, prevalence increased with age and was more common in women (10% vs. 5%), but not all studies provided information on gender or age. Frailty was also more common when defined using the frailty index rather than the phenotype approach (14% vs. 10%).

A number of studies have been published since the 2012 review. One study using Fried criteria in a sample of 511 over-64s from a St Petersburg district reported an overall prevalence of 21%, 63%, and 16% for frailty, pre-frailty, and non-frailty, respectively (29). Using the Steverink-Slaets model (30) and the extended Puts model (31), researchers found the prevalence of frailty to be 33% and 44%, respectively. The authors also reported that the Fried model had the highest association with dependency. The Garre-Olmo study mentioned earlier reported that 39% of the over-75 population demonstrated one or more of three types of frailty (18); values for physical, mental, and social frailty were 17%, 20%, and 9%, respectively (some people exhibited two or three of the phenotypes). In an even older population of 86-year-old community-dwelling individuals, the prevalence of frailty was 20%, with 54% pre-frail and 25% non-frail using the Fried criteria (32). Finally, a Dutch study of 102 primary care patients over 65 years (33) reported frailty rates of 12 to 36% using seven different scales.

5 **Frailty and sarcopenia**

Low muscle mass together with either low muscle strength or low physical performance have been suggested as the criteria for sarcopenia (34). The latter two features are also contained within the Fried criteria; not surprisingly, there is overlap between the two conditions. An analysis of data from the Aging and Longevity Study (35) showed that the presence of sarcopenia increased the risk of all causes of death in over-80s, with a hazard ratio of 2.32. It is still to be determined whether identifying this sub-group of patients has any benefit in terms of identifying people at risk of adverse health outcomes or indicating specific treatments. Patients with dementia, which is also a wasting disease, meet phenotype criteria for frailty as well. The relationship between these two conditions has been discussed (4).

6 **Treatment of frailty**

Frailty has the features of a 'geriatric giant' as originally defined by Isaacs (36). Among the cardinal features of the giants are the complexity of the condition, the multiple causes, and the absence of a single straightforward treatment. So it is with the frailty syndrome no matter how defined. Although anabolic steroids and anti-inflammatory treatments have been suggested (37), at the present time there are no recognized specific pharmaceutical treatments for the frailty syndrome itself—just treatments for individual diseases that contribute to it. Table 7.2 lists some common conditions associated with frailty along with possible interventions. Patients who are frail are often excluded from clinical trials, so that even for common diseases the value of treatment for frail patients is not clear (38, 39). Indeed, Jeffery et al. (40) suggest that treating frail hypertensive patients may be detrimental, as it has been reported that in those with the slowest walking speeds a higher blood pressure appeared to be protective of mortality (41). This issue is discussed further by Hubbard et al. (42).

7 **Recent developments and future trends**

7.1 **Developments in primary care**

Until recently the study of frailty has been the domain of geriatricians and epidemiologists, although, of course, the majority of frail older people will have their health care needs met by primary care physicians and their teams. Lacas and Rockwood drew attention to the shortage of geriatricians worldwide and highlighted the imperative for primary care physicians to identify which of their patients are frail (43). However, it has not yet been established which tools are best to do this. Hoogendijk and colleagues (33) compared a number of scales against Fried criteria and expert panel consensus in general practice.

Table 7.2 Disorders that may lead to increasing frailty including possible treatments

Condition/Disorder	Treatment
Blood clotting activity	Aspirin
Anaemia	Haematinic replacement therapy
	Recombinant human erythropoietin
Arthritis	NSAIDs
	Steroids
CHD	Antihypertensives
	Aspirin
	Statins
Cognitive impairment	Cholinesterase inhibitors
	Exercise
Depression	Exercise
	Social interaction
	Counselling
	Psychotherapy
	Antidepressants
Falls/fractures	Vitamin D
	Calcium treatment
	Exercise
Hypothyroidism	L-thyroxine
Increased blood clotting activity	Aspirin
Inflammation/muscle strength	Exercise
	Statins/ACE inhibitors
Lowered testosterone (males)	Replacement therapy
Poor nutrition	Dietary regulation
Type 2 diabetes	Thiazolidinedione
	Antiglycaemics

They found that the simple questionnaire approach of PRISMA-7 (44) produced better sensitivity and specificity than the standard Fried criteria and that of an expert panel. Its clinical utility remains to be determined, however.

The collection of additional data over and above what is obtained as part of routine primary care obviously causes additional work. The potential for using routinely collected data was explored by Drubbel et al. (45). They constructed a frailty index based on some of the data items collected by the International Classification of Primary Care routine health care data plus an additional item on polypharmacy. Their 36-item frailty index predicted adverse health outcomes: 43% of those in the highest tertile developed an adverse health outcome compared to 12% in the lowest tertile. However, the clinical usefulness of this approach has not been established.

An interesting development in this area is the potential of frailty measurements to facilitate inter-professional management, so that members of the team can have a common understanding of any individual's status and risk. It has been suggested that the clinical global impression of change in physical frailty (46), the Edmonton Frailty Scale (47), and the Dynamic Frailty scale (31) may all be useful in this situation (48).

7.2 **Future trends**

Since there is still no consensus on the definition of frailty, but recognition that one is needed, it is probable that articles will continue to be published advocating new or modified methodologies. The ultimate candidate has to be generally accepted and be:

- proven in good-quality clinical trials
- simple and quick enough for clinicians to use as part of their normal practice.
- predictive.

The emphasis in the literature is on finding a treatment for frailty. However, since frailty is complex and heterogeneous in nature, the most likely successful interventions will be those that identify the underlying diseases and treat them. Other than this, numerous studies on geriatric syndromes in general, and frailty in particular, espouse the beneficial effects of exercise.

The interest in inflammatory and immunological predictors of frailty is growing. There are now several population studies that are looking for specific biological markers of frailty in older adults. In addition, animal models of frailty can test various hypotheses and explore potential genetic and/or environmental stimuli that increase or decrease the risk of becoming frail.

Interest is also growing in possible vaccinations that may prevent frailty. A possible treatment approach is to vaccinate young adults when the immune system is uncompromised. Potential vaccinations could be against viruses such as CMV to prevent them accessing and lying dormant within cells. Testing has also begun on vaccines with greater immunogenicity to replace the current flu vaccines in frail or pre-frail older adults. In this way a strong immune memory can be built up that may prevent individuals getting influenza.

8 **Conclusion**

Despite the lack of a standard definition and uncertainty of frailty's role in the classification of disease it looks as if the term is here to stay. The Department of Health in England has appointed its first National Clinical Director for

Integration and Frail Elderly. However, in this service-delivery context the term encompasses both those who meet diagnostic criteria for a frailty phenotype as well as all other older people with complex chronic needs and multiple morbidities.

As well as a lack of clarity over definition there is a lack of clarity over the purpose of using the term. As a predictor of adverse outcome it is insufficiently predictive (49). If a person has a severe single-system disease such as heart failure or cancer, one does not need a frailty index or phenotype judgement to determine that there is a risk of death. Prediction of institutionalization is a more complex issue, however. It depends not only on the state of the individual but also on the availability of care homes, the support available at home, and the psychological state of the older person and their family. Identification of people who might benefit from a specific anti-frailty pharmaceutical therapy seems distant, although targeting the sarcopenia type of frailty might be more promising. Therefore at the moment detection of frailty would seem best an epidemiological tool and an adjuvant way of identifying those at risk.

Websites relevant to this chapter

Canadian Initiative on Frailty and Aging:

<http://www.frail-fragile.ca/e/index.htm>

The King's Fund (various frailty topics):

<http://www.kingsfund.org.uk/search/site/frail>

References

1 **Chambers 21st century dictionary**. Edinburgh: Chambers; 1999. p. 525.
2 **Gilleard C, Higgs P**. Frailty, disability and old age: a re-appraisal. Health. 2011;**15**(5):475–90.
3 **Woodhouse KW, Wynne HILA, Baillie SHEL, James OFW, Rawlins MD**. Who are the frail elderly? Q J Med, 1988. **68**(1):505–6.
4 **Sampson EL**. Frailty and dementia: common but complex comorbidities. Aging Ment Health. 2012;**16**(3):269–72. doi: 10.1080/13607863.2012.657158. Epub 2012 Mar 2.
5 **McLachlan AJ, Bath S, Naganathan V, Hilmer SN, Le Couteur DG, et al**. Clinical pharmacology of analgesic medicines in older people: impact of frailty and cognitive impairment. Br J Clin Pharmacol. 2011;**71**(3):351–64. doi: 10.1111/j.1365-2125.2010.03847.x
6 **Rockwood K, Song X, MacKnight C, Bergman H, Hogan DB, et al**. A global clinical measure of fitness and frailty in elderly people. Can Med Assoc J. 2005;**173**(5):489–95.
7 **Rodriguez-Manas L, Feart C, Mann G, Vina J, Chatterji S, et al**. Searching for an operational definition of frailty: a Delphi method based consensus statement: the frailty operative definition-consensus conference project. J Gerontol A-Biol. 2013;**68**(1):62–7.

8 Fried LP, Tangen CM, Walston J, Newman AB, Hirsch C, et al. Frailty in older adults: evidence for a phenotype. J Gerontol A-Biol. 2001;56(3):M146-M157.

9 Wou F, Conroy S. The frailty syndrome. Medicine. 2013;41(1):13-5.

10 Bandeen-Roche K, Xue QL, Ferrucci L, Walston J, Guralnik JM, et al. Phenotype of frailty: characterization in the Women's Health and Aging studies. J Gerontol A-Biol. 2006;61(3):262-6.

11 Ensrud KE, Ewing SK, Cawthon PM, Fink HA, Taylor BC, et al. A comparison of frailty indexes for the prediction of falls, disability, fractures, and mortality in older men. J Am Geriatr Soc. 2009;57(3):492-8.

12 Montesanto A, Lagani V, Martino C, Dato S, De Rango F, et al. A novel, population-specific approach to define frailty. AGE. 2010;32(3):385-95.

13 Mitnitski AB, Mogilner AJ, Rockwood K. Accumulation of deficits as a proxy measure of aging. Sci World J. 2001;1:323-36.

14 Searle SD, Mitnitski A, Gahbauer EA, Gill TM, Rockwood K. A standard procedure for creating a frailty index. BMC Geriatr. 2008;8:24. doi: 10.1186/1471-2318-8-24

15 Romero-Ortuno R, Kenny RA. The frailty index in Europeans: association with age and mortality. Age Ageing. 2012;41(5):684-9. doi: 10.1093/ageing/afs051. Epub 2012 Apr 19.

16 Romero-Ortuno R, O'Shea D, Kenny RA. The SHARE frailty instrument for primary care predicts incident disability in a European population-based sample. Qual Prim Care. 2011;19(5):301-9.

17 Hubbard RE, Theou O. Frailty: enhancing the known knowns. Age Ageing. 2012;41(5):574-5. doi: 10.1093/ageing/afs093. Epub 2012 Jul 10.

18 Garre-Olmo J, Calvo-Perxas L, Lopez-Pousa S, de Gracia Blanco M, Vilalta-Franch J. Prevalence of frailty phenotypes and risk of mortality in a community-dwelling elderly cohort. Age Ageing. 2013;42(1):46-51. doi: 10.1093/ageing/afs047. Epub 2012 Mar 27.

19 Parks RJ, Fares E, Macdonald JK, Ernst MC, Sinal CJ, et al. A procedure for creating a frailty index based on deficit accumulation in aging mice. J Gerontol A-Biol. 2012;67(3):217-27. doi: 10.1093/gerona/glr193. Epub 2011 Oct 21.

20 Schmaltz HN, Fried LP, Xue QL, Walston J, Leng SX, et al. Chronic cytomegalovirus infection and inflammation are associated with prevalent frailty in community-dwelling older women. J Amer Ger Soc. 2005;53(5):747-754.

21 Wang GC, Kao WHL, Murakami P, Xue Q-L, Chiou RB, Detrick B, McDyer JF, Semba RD, Casolaro V, Walston JD, et al. Cytomegalovirus infection and the risk of mortality and frailty in older women: a prospective observational cohort study. Amer J Epidemiol. 2010;171:1144-52.

22 Baylis D, Bartlett D, Syddall H, Ntani G, Gale C, et al. Immune-endocrine biomarkers as predictors of frailty and mortality: a 10-year longitudinal study in community-dwelling older people. AGE. 2013;35(3):963-71.

23 Haeseker MB, Pijpers E, Dukers-Muijrers NH, Nelemans P, Hoebe CJ, et al. Association of cytomegalovirus and other pathogens with frailty and diabetes mellitus, but not with cardiovascular disease and mortality in psycho-geriatric patients; a prospective cohort study. Immun Ageing. 2013;10(1):30.

24 Li H, Manwani B, Leng SX. Frailty inflammation, and immunity. Aging Dis. 2011;2(6):466-73. Epub 2011 Dec 2.

25 Le Saux S, Weyand CM, Goronzy JJ. Mechanisms of immunosenescence: lessons from models of accelerated immune aging. Ann NY Acad Sci. 2012;**1247**(1):69–82.

26 McElhaney JE, Zhou X, Talbot HK, Soethout E, Bleackley RC, et al. The unmet need in the elderly: how immunosenescence, CMV infection, co-morbidities and frailty are a challenge for the development of more effective influenza vaccines. Vaccine. 2012;**30**(12):2060–7. doi: 10.1016/j.vaccine.2012.01.015. Epub 2012 Jan 27.

27 Salvioli S, Monti D, Lanzarini C, Conte M, Pirazzini C, et al. Immune system, cell senescence, aging and longevity—inflammaging reappraised. Curr Pharm Des. 2013;**19**(9):1675–9.

28 Collard RM, Boter H, Schoevers RA, Oude Voshaar RC. Prevalence of frailty in community-dwelling older persons: a systematic review. J Am Geriatr Soc. 2012;**60**(8): 1487–92. doi: 10.1111/j.1532–5415.2012.04054.x. Epub 2012 Aug 6.

29 Gurina NA, Frolova EV, Degryse JM, A roadmap of aging in Russia: the prevalence of frailty in community-dwelling older adults in the St. Petersburg district—the 'Crystal' study. J Am Geriatr Soc. 2011;**59**(6):980–8. doi: 10.1111/j.1532–5415.2011.03448.x. Epub 2011 Jun 7.

30 Steverink N, Slaets JPJ, Schuurmans H, Lis MV. Measuring frailty: development and testing of the Groningen Frailty Indicator (GFI). Gerontologist. 2001;**41**(Special issue 1):236–7.

31 Puts MT, Lips P, Deeg DJ. Static and dynamic measures of frailty predicted decline in performance-based and self-reported physical functioning. J Clin Epidemiol. 2005;**58**(11):1188–98.

32 Ferrer A, Badia T, Formiga F, Sanz H, Megido MJ, et al. Frailty in the oldest old: prevalence and associated factors. J Am Geriatr Soc. 2013;**61**(2):294–6. doi: 10.1111/jgs.12154

33 Hoogendijk EO, van der Horst HE, Deeg DJ, Frijters DH, Prins BA, et al. The identification of frail older adults in primary care: comparing the accuracy of five simple instruments. Age Ageing. 2013;**42**(2):262–5. doi: 10.1093/ageing/afs163. Epub 2012 Oct 28.

34 Cruz-Jentoft AJ, Baeyens JP, Bauer JRM, Boirie Y, Cederholm T, et al. Sarcopenia: European consensus on definition and diagnosis. Age Ageing. 2010;**39**(4):412–23.

35 Landi F, Cruz-Jentoft AJ, Liperoti R, Russo A, Giovannini S, et al. Sarcopenia and mortality risk in frail older persons aged 80 years and older: results from ilSIRENTE study. Age Ageing. 2013;**42**(2):203–9. doi: 10.1093/ageing/afs194. Epub 2013 Jan 15.

36 Crome P, Lally F. Frailty: joining the giants. Can Med Assoc J, 2011. **183**(8):889–90.

37 Walston J, Hadley EC, Ferrucci L, Guralnik JM, Newman AB, et al. Research agenda for frailty in older adults: toward a better understanding of physiology and etiology: summary from the American Geriatrics Society/National Institute on Aging Research Conference on Frailty in Older Adults. J Am Geriatr Soc. 2006;**54**(6):991–1001.

38 Cherubini A, Oristrell J, Pla X, et al. The persistent exclusion of older patients from ongoing clinical trials regarding heart failure. Arch Intern Med. 2011;**171**(6):550–6.

39 Crome P, Lally F, Cherubini A, Oristrell J, Beswick AD, et al. Exclusion of older people from clinical trials: professional views from nine European countries participating in the PREDICT study. Drugs Aging. 2011;**28**(8):667–77. doi: 10.2165/11591990–000000000–00000

40 Jeffery CA, Shum DW, Hubbard RE. Emerging drug therapies for frailty. Maturitas. 2013;**74**(1):21–5. doi: 10.1016/j.maturitas.2012.10.010. Epub 2012 Nov 7.

41 Odden MC, Peralta CA, Haan MN, Covinsky KE. Rethinking the association of high blood pressure with mortality in elderly adults: the impact of frailty. Arch Intern Med. 2012;**172**(15):1162–8. doi: 10.1001/archinternmed.2012.2555

42 Hubbard RE, O'Mahony MS, Woodhouse KW. Medication prescribing in frail older people. Eur J Clin Pharmacol. 2013;**69**(3):319–26. doi: 10.1007/s00228-012-1387-2. Epub 2012 Sep 11.

43 Lacas A, Rockwood K. Frailty in primary care: a review of its conceptualization and implications for practice. BMC Med. 2012;**10**:4.(doi):10.1186/1741-7015-10-4

44 Raiche M, Hebert R, Dubois MF. PRISMA-7: a case-finding tool to identify older adults with moderate to severe disabilities. Arch Gerontol Geriatr. 2008;**47**(1):9–18. Epub 2007 Aug 27.

45 Drubbel I, de Wit NJ, Bleijenberg N, Eijkemans RJ, Schuurmans MJ, et al. Prediction of adverse health outcomes in older people using a frailty index based on routine primary care data. J Gerontol A-Biol. 2013;**68**(3):301–8. doi: 10.1093/gerona/gls161. Epub 2012 Jul 25.

46 Studenski S, Hayes RP, Leibowitz RQ, Bode R, Lavery L, et al. Clinical global impression of change in physical frailty: development of a measure based on clinical judgment. J Am Geriatr Soc. 2004;**52**(9):1560–6.

47 Rolfson DB, Majumdar SR, Tsuyuki RT, Tahir A, Rockwood K. Validity and reliability of the Edmonton Frail Scale. Age Ageing. 2006;**35**(5):526–9.

48 Poltawski L, Goodman C, Iliffe S, Manthorpe J, Gage H, et al. Frailty scales—their potential in interprofessional working with older people: a discussion paper. J Interprof Care. 2011;**25**(4):280–6. doi: 10.3109/13561820.2011.562332. Epub 2011 May 9.

49 Daniels R, van Rossum E, Beurskens A, van den Heuvel W, de Witte L. The predictive validity of three self-report screening instruments for identifying frail older people in the community. BMC Public Health. 2012;**12**:69.

Chapter 8

Incontinence, the sleeping geriatric giant: challenges and solutions

Adrian Wagg

Key points

- The prevalence of urinary incontinence increases in association with increasing age.
- Behavioural and lifestyle interventions, including exercise, are effective in older people.
- There is an increasing evidence base for pharmacological therapy of urgency incontinence in the elderly and frail elderly.
- Surgical management for older men and women is associated with benefit but should be performed with due regard to potential benefits and harms, remaining life expectancy, and the expectations of both patient and, where relevant, caregiver.
- Continence care should ideally be based around provision by specialist nurse practitioners working within a multiprofessional, integrated service.

1 Introduction

The maintenance of continence is a basic human function, partially dependent upon intact lower urinary tract function, but also on the necessary cerebral control, not only of urination but of social appropriateness of actions, mobility, and dexterity. Continence remains a little talked about subject for many older people and 'bladder problems or weakness' are often thought of as a necessary part of growing older. Urinary incontinence (UI) is certainly not a part of normal ageing although lower urinary tract symptoms are highly prevalent in later life. Urinary incontinence, in a similar fashion to other problems in late life, reflects a typical geriatric syndrome, with multiple risk and modulating factors acting together to produce an end effect. Thus, urinary incontinence is as much a diagnosis as is one of 'falls' or 'delirium', and effort needs to be made to identify the underlying factors which contribute to the problem. Such complexity should not be unduly daunting. Geriatricians are well used to the complexity paradigm in the context of falls and cognitive impairment; incontinence in older people is no different.

2 Prevalence and relation to age-associated changes in the brain

The prevalence of urinary incontinence increases with increasing age, affecting approximately 11% of men and 20% of women over the age of 60 (1). In addition to usual lower urinary tract pathology, incontinence in later life is perhaps dominated by an increasing inability to inhibit voiding in response to the sensation of urge to void. Investigation of older people with urgency has revealed an increased load of white matter hyperintensities in those with symptomatic urgency and difficulty in maintaining continence. These findings also link incontinence with cognitive and functional impairment, which may be a final common pathway in the generation of late-life geriatric syndromes (2).

3 Types of incontinence

3.1 Urgency and urgency incontinence

Urinary urgency is the hallmark symptom of overactive bladder (OAB), which for approximately a third of adults is associated with urgency urinary incontinence (3). The prevalence and incidence of urgency and urgency incontinence increases with age. In the EPIC (European Prospective Investigation into Cancer and Nutrition) study of adults over 40, based upon a structured telephone interview of more than 19,000 people, 19.1% (95% CI: 17.5–20.7) community-dwelling men and 18.3% (16.9–19.6) women over the age of 60 indicated that they had urinary urgency, and 2.5% (1.9–3.1) men and 2.5% (1.9–3.0) women indicated that they had urgency incontinence (1). More recently, reports from longitudinal studies in cohorts of men and women have illustrated the age-related increase in lower urinary tract symptoms, including urgency and urgency incontinence. In the study of women, 2,911 women responded to a self-administered postal questionnaire in 1991 and 1,408 of the women replied to the same survey in 2007. Over that time, the prevalence of UI, OAB, and nocturia increased by 13%, 9%, and 20%, respectively. The proportion of women with OAB and UUI increased from 6% to 16% (4). In men (5), 7,763 responded to a self-administered postal questionnaire in 1992, and 3,257 responded to the same survey in 2009. In a similar fashion, prevalence of UI and OAB increased (overall UI from 4.5% to 10.5%; OAB from 15.6% to 44.4%). The prevalence of nocturia, urgency, slow stream, hesitancy, incomplete emptying, postmicturition dribble, and daytime frequency also increased.

3.2 **Stress urinary incontinence**

Stress urinary incontinence (SUI), urinary loss which occurs on exertion or effort, appears to have its peak incidence in women in mid-life. In the EPIC study (1), 8.0% (95% CI: 7.1–9.0) of women over 60 had the condition. In men, the majority of SUI occurs following prostatic surgery, with rates varying depending upon the type of operation. Transurethral resection of the prostate is associated with rates of approximately 1% (6), whereas retropubic radical prostatectomy is associated with rates between 2% and 57% (7, 8), depending upon selection, definition, and time frame, but the proportion of men with SUI is generally more prevalent in the oldest groups. EPIC revealed a prevalence of 5.2% (95% CI: 4.2–6.1) in men over 60 years of age.

3.3 **Mixed urinary incontinence**

Although there are operational difficulties with the definition of mixed incontinence, particularly in cystometric terms, when regarded as urinary incontinence with symptoms of both urinary urgency incontinence and exertional incontinence, mixed incontinence is highly prevalent in primary care (9). To what extent this finding reflects uncertainty in history-taking (in that severe urethral sphincter incompetence can produce a feeling of precipitant urinary loss at pressure threshold or as urine enters the bladder neck and is reported as urgency), is unclear. Some epidemiological data suggest that mixed incontinence accounts for approximately one third of all cases of incontinence in women. Even so, mixed urinary incontinence accounted for only 4.1% of incontinence in women over 60 years of age in the EPIC study, probably highlighting the difficulty with the operational definition (1, 10).

3.4 **Nocturnal enuresis**

Whereas nocturia is extremely common in older people, nocturnal enuresis is less so. In a study of 3,884 community-dwelling men and women aged 65 to 79, nocturnal enuresis was reported by 2.1%, and was significantly higher among women (2.9%) than men (11). It is often accompanied by other associated lower urinary tract symptoms and complicated by associated co-morbid conditions or the effects of medications affecting sleep. Congestive heart failure, functional disability, depression, nocturnal polyuria, and use of hypnotics at least once per week have been associated with the condition. Adult-onset nocturnal enuresis without daytime symptoms in an older person without significant co-morbidity is a serious symptom. Usually it is a sign of significant urological pathology and should be thoroughly investigated (12).

3.5 Functional incontinence

Urinary incontinence in older people may be wholly unrelated to lower urinary tract abnormality. Successful toileting requires sufficient cognitive and physical function, including manual dexterity, to reach the toilet, undress, and void in a timely and socially appropriate fashion. For many frail older people, the burden of either physical or cognitive impairment renders this less likely. Incontinence in these situations is termed functional. There is little systematic evaluation or assessment of either the prevalence or management of this clinical entity. Much that is practised is as a result of received wisdom, involving lifestyle and behavioural techniques employed for the general management of incontinence in frail older people.

4 Voiding inefficiency

The finding of a post-voiding residual volume of urine is far from uncommon in an older population. In one survey of community-dwelling men and women over age 75, more than 10 ml of residual urine was found in 91 of the 92 men (median 90 ml; range 10–1502 ml) and in 44 of the 48 women (median 45 ml; range 0–180 ml) (13). In a study of men undergoing urological work-up, the finding of a post-void residual greater than 50 ml was 2.5 times greater for men with a prostate volume greater than 30 ml than in those with smaller prostates. Men with a post-void residual greater than 50 ml were about three times as likely to have subsequent acute urinary retention with catheterization during the subsequent three to four years (14). A separate study in older women found a residual volume of 100mL or more in up to 10% of older women, many of whom were asymptomatic. It appeared that the residual volume remitted over a two-year period (15). It is evident that there is a reduction in the contractile function of the bladder associated with ageing in both men and women. Probably this is due to a dampening of detrusor contractile force by the age-associated accumulation of surrounding connective tissue (16, 17). What constitutes a normal post-void residual in older people is still widely debated; the common concerns about recurrent urinary tract infection, incontinence, and upper renal tract damage are not well substantiated in otherwise normal older people, the risk of high pressures being low (18). There is no effective pharmacological therapy for ineffective voiding and, in the absence of outflow tract obstruction, no effective surgical intervention. Management consists of double voiding; if this proves ineffective then catheterization, either intermittent or indwelling, is the treatment of choice.

5 Quality of life and impact

The impact of incontinence in older people is often described in terms of its association with other conditions: UI is associated with an increased risk of falls and fracture, urinary tract infection, depression, and skin problems, and is an independent risk for institutionalization (19–21). In a large population-based observation study, UI (defined as use of pads) was independently associated with one other geriatric condition (of cognitive impairment, injurious falls, dizziness, vision impairment, or hearing impairment) in 60%, two or more conditions in 28%, and three or more in 13% (22). Associated conditions such as peripheral vascular disease, Parkinson's disease (PD), diabetes mellitus, congestive heart failure, venous insufficiency and chronic lung disease, falls and contractures, recurrent infection and constipation have all been implicated in generating a predisposition to the development of UI (Table 8.1).

Hypertension, congestive heart failure, arthritis, depression, and anxiety were associated with a higher prevalence of UI. A linear correlation ($r = 0.81$) was found between prevalence of UI and the number of co-morbid conditions (23). Moreover, incontinence has an impact on the quality of life and well-being of older people, leading to reduced socialization, associated with the severity of the incontinence, rather than the type, although other studies suggest that urgency incontinence has a greater impact than the other subtypes (24–26). There are also data to suggest a reduction in economic productivity and increased work absence for those with incontinence (27). While not immediately relevant, as the requirement for people to remain economically active until later in life increases, this is likely to become an important factor. The additional impact on informal caregivers of those with incontinence is also significant in terms of burden and reduced quality of life (28). The economic impact of some of those caregivers leaving the workforce to care for older people with incontinence has not been quantified. However, the additional costs associated with OAB and related incontinence in the UK has been estimated at €515 per year per patient, with nursing home continence care accounting for an additional €381 per year above that amount, the majority of this relating to containment products (29).

Table 8.1 Co-morbid medications associated with urinary incontinence in older people

Conditions	Comments	Implications for Management
Co-morbid medical illnesses Diabetes mellitus Degenerative joint disease Chronic pulmonary disease Congestive heart failure Lower extremity venous insufficiency Sleep apnoea	Poor control can cause polyuria and precipitate or exacerbate incontinence; also associated with increased likelihood of urgency incontinence and diabetic neuropathic bladder Can impair mobility and precipitate urgency UI Associated cough can worsen stress UI Increased night-time urine production can contribute to nocturia and UI May increase night-time urine production by increasing production of atrial natriuretic peptide	Better control of diabetes can reduce osmotic diuresis and associated polyuria, and improve incontinence Optimal pharmacologic and non-pharmacologic pain management can improve mobility and toileting ability Cough suppression can reduce stress incontinence and cough-induced urgency UI Optimizing pharmacologic management of congestive heart failure, sodium restriction, support stockings, leg elevation, and a late afternoon dose of a rapid-acting diuretic may reduce nocturnal polyuria and associated nocturia and night-time UI Diagnosis and treatment of sleep apnoea, usually with continuous positive airway pressure devices, may improve the condition and reduce nocturnal polyuria and associated nocturia and UI
Severe constipation and faecal impaction	Associated with 'double' incontinence (urinary and faecal)	Appropriate use of stool softeners Adequate fluid intake and exercise Disimpaction if necessary

Table 8.1 (continued) Co-morbid medications associated with urinary incontinence in older people

Conditions	Comments	Implications for Management
Neurological and psychiatric conditions Stroke Parkinson's disease Normal pressure hydrocephalus Dementia (Alzheimer's, multi-infarct, others) Depression	Can precipitate urgency UI and less often urinary retention; also impairs mobility Associated with urgency UI; also causes impaired mobility and cognition in late stages Presents with UI, along with gait and cognitive impairments Associated with urgency UI; impaired cognition and apraxia interferes with toileting and hygiene May impair motivation to be continent; may also be a consequence of incontinence	UI after an acute stroke often resolves with rehabilitation; persistent UI should be further evaluated Regular toileting assistance essential for those with persistent mobility impairment Optimizing management may improve mobility and improve UI Regular toileting assistance essential for those with mobility and cognitive impairment in late stages Patients presenting with all three symptoms should be considered for brain imaging to rule out this condition, as it may improve with a ventricular-peritoneal shunt Regular toileting assistance essential for those with mobility and cognitive impairment in late stages Optimizing pharmacological and non-pharmacological management of depression may improve UI
Medications	See Table 8.2	Discontinuation or modification of drug regimen
Functional impairments Impaired mobility Impaired cognition	Impaired cognition and/or mobility due to a variety of conditions listed above and others can interfere with the ability to toilet independently and precipitate UI	Regular toileting assistance essential for those with severe mobility and/or cognitive impairment
Environmental factors Inaccessible toilets Unsafe toilet facilities Unavailable caregivers for toileting assistance	Frail, functionally impaired persons require accessible, safe toilet facilities, and in many cases human assistance in order to be continent	Environmental alterations may be helpful; supportive measures such as pads may be necessary if caregiver assistance is not regularly available

6 Evidence base for treatment

The evidence base for treatment of the elderly, specifically the frail elderly, lags behind that for community-dwelling adults. The difficulty of recruiting the elderly to clinical studies is well recognized (30) and is compounded by multiple exclusion criteria, meaning that the majority of older people become ineligible for study even if willing and able to participate. Despite the high prevalence of the condition and the increased severity experienced by older people, they tend to be excluded from treatment trials of pharmacotherapy and surgery. Data do however exist for conservative and prompted voiding and functional incidental training (exercise) in nursing home residents. The usefulness of this technique (and others like it) is limited by both the intensity of the intervention in relation to available staff time and perhaps more so recently by the changing demographics of those admitted to nursing home care, where 60% have a dementia diagnosis and 40% lose their mobility within six months of admission. The guidelines for care of frail older people within the International Consultation on Incontinence (published 2013) contains the most up-to-date synthesis of available evidence concerning conservative and behavioural interventions (31).

7 Treatment strategies for treating incontinence in the elderly

7.1 Lifestyle interventions

Several lifestyle interventions have been evaluated in healthier older women, including dieting and medication to help with weight loss, fluid selection (caffeine, alcohol, and volume), and constipation management. There are much fewer data in healthier older men and almost no data on frail older people (32). The international consultation on incontinence referred to earlier took the view that should there be evidence of efficacy for any intervention in a general population of older people, then it would seem unreasonable not to offer that intervention to the frail elderly, given that the intervention was feasible and congruent with the aims of management and expectations of that person (31). A trial of caffeine restriction, for example, may superficially result in little harm, but may adversely affect the hydration status of an older person for little perceived benefit.

7.2 Behavioural interventions

Behavioural interventions have been especially designed for frail older people with cognitive and physical impairments. Because these behavioural interventions have no side effects, they have been the mainstay of UI treatment in frail older people (33). The technique with the most evidence for its use is *prompted voiding*. Subjects are prompted to use the lavatory and encouraged with social reward when successfully toileted. This technique increases patient requests for toileting and self-initiated toileting, and decreases the number of UI episodes (34). A three-day trial during which the number of incontinent episodes should reduce by 20% would be considered successful. The second commonly used technique, *habit retraining*, requires the identification of the incontinent person's individual toileting pattern and UI episodes, usually by means of a bladder diary. A toileting schedule is then devised to pre-empt them (35, 36). *Timed voiding* involves toileting at fixed intervals, such as every three hours. There is no patient education, reinforcement of behaviours, or attempt to re-establish normal voiding patterns (37).

7.3 Functional incidental training

Functional incidental training incorporates musculoskeletal strengthening exercises into toileting routines by nursing home care aides (nursing assistants) (38).

There is increasing evidence for the effectiveness of physical exercise as an intervention for urinary incontinence in populations in diverse settings. In a veterans nursing home population in the United States, the combination of prompted voiding and individualized, functionally oriented endurance and strengthening exercises offered four times per day, five days per week, for eight weeks was effective in significantly reducing urinary incontinence (39). An intervention which provided exercise and incontinence care every two hours from 8:00 a.m. to 4:30 p.m. (total of four daily care episodes) for five days a week over 32 weeks in a nursing home population was also found to be effective in significantly reducing incontinence (40). Similarly, a study of walking exercise for thirty minutes per day in a small group of cognitively impaired residents over four weeks resulted in a significant reduction in daytime incontinence episodes and an increase in gait speed and stamina (41). A 30-minute intervention conducted by allied health professionals three times weekly over eight weeks proved effective in increasing the number of subjects who achieved independent toileting but did not significantly reduce daily urine loss (42). In community-dwelling older people, a 30-minute evening walk proved effective in reducing nocturia, while also improving daytime urinary frequency, blood pressure, body weight, body fat ratio, triglycerides, total cholesterol, and sleep quality (43). Cognitive and functional impairment, common in frail elderly people, may preclude the use of some of these interventions. Additionally, the context in which care is provided needs to be considered (44–46). Many of these interventions are time-consuming and need effective staff engagement to deliver effectively (47).

Although pelvic floor muscle training (PFMT) has not been studied extensively in frail older people, age and frailty alone should not preclude its use in patients with sufficient cognition to participate. An intervention involving information about urinary function combined with bladder training was effective among community-dwelling women aged between 55 and 80 years (48). The women were provided with the following information: slides and handouts about normal lower urinary tract anatomy and function; types of incontinence; effects of incontinence on lifestyle; healthy habits and self-care. The women were also given instruction and practice in bladder training and pelvic floor muscle training (PFMT), and how to incorporate these into everyday activities. The PFMT instructions—delivered via audiotape—suggested daily practice as well as bladder training if the intervoid interval was less than 3.5 hours. The fact that the programme was successful for this sample of women suggests it may be as well for older women who are frail.

7.4 Pharmacological therapy

The main target for pharmacological therapy of UI associated with storage symptoms is OAB/urgency-frequency syndrome. Here, antimuscarinic drugs are the mainstay of treatment. There is accumulating evidence—perhaps because of the increased severity of UI in older people, or because they are less successful with behavioural or lifestyle measures—that they are not only more likely to request drug therapy to control their OAB symptoms if medication is withdrawn (49), but are more likely to need higher doses of drug to achieve most benefit, particularly in the oldest old (>75 years) (50, 51). Additionally, older people appear to be more adherent to their therapy than the young (52).

Data on the efficacy of antimuscarinic agents in community-dwelling older people exist from both *post hoc*, pooled analyses from registration trials of antimuscarinic agents and, increasingly, from trials specifically designed to assess the efficacy of newer agents in the older population. There are fewer data about the use of such agents in older men and in older frailer individuals. One study of extended release oxybutynin examines cognitive effects in nursing home residents with dementia and urgency UI (53). Published trials of the efficacy of transdermal oxybutynin included subjects up to age 100 and those in institutional care settings, but did not stratify results by age or co-morbidity (54). Fesoterodine has been studied in older people identified as frail by the Vulnerable Elders Survey (55). There are data on the comparative pharmacokinetics short term efficacy and longer term safety of mirabegron, an FDA-approved beta-3 agonist, in older people but not specifically in the frail elderly. In available pharmacokinetic studies, there were no statistically significant differences in mirabegron exposure between older (55 years and above) and younger (18–45 years) volunteers. Similar results were obtained for those aged 65 years and above. The area under the curve for exposure was predicted to be 11% higher in a subject 90 years of age.

Overall, pharmacological therapy in older people should be considered in the same light as other therapies and doses started low for tolerability, rather than efficacy concerns. Meta-analysis suggests that the efficacy of each drug in relieving the symptoms of OAB and improving quality of life is essentially comparable. Responses to commonly used antimuscarinics from available studies which report on older people are shown in Table 8.2. The most common side effects of antimuscarinics are dry mouth and constipation, which may limit their use on some older people. A network meta-analysis illustrates the relative incidence of side effects in a comparative method (56). There is evidence that treatment is not associated with either falls or delirium, often cited by geriatricians as a reason not to treat UI with antimuscarinic drugs (57, 58).

Newer medications, such as the beta-3 agonist mirabegron, have also been shown to be effective in community-dwelling elderly, but only in a pooled analysis from available registration trials (66). The side-effect profile of immediate release oral oxybutynin and its potential for subclinical cognitive impairment in those cognitively at risk, particularly at high doses, mitigates against its use in older people. The newer antimuscarinics each have a place in management, and physicians should be confident in using these, increasing the dose where necessary and swapping them should there be inefficacy. There are data on the cognitive effects of bladder antimuscarinics (darifenacin, fesoterodine, solifenacin, tolterodine, transdermal oxybutynin gel, trospium chloride) in cognitively intact older people and for solifenacin in older people with mild cognitive impairment (67–73). The quaternary ammonium compound trospium chloride does not cross the elderly blood-brain barrier and has a low potential for drug-drug interactions. The drugs darifenacin and 5-hydroxymethyl tolterodine penetrate the blood-brain barrier but are substrates for p-glycoproteins, and are actively transported from the central nervous system. Transdermal preparations of oxybutynin are associated with low levels of antimuscarinic side effects.

7.5 **Pharmacological therapy for nocturia**

Nocturia is highly prevalent among the elderly. Typically nocturia of two or more nightly episodes is associated with a significant impact on quality of life. Additionally, some studies have associated nocturia with falls in the elderly, increased mortality, and early development of coronary vascular disease. Nocturia may also be associated with bladder outflow tract obstruction and OAB. Most patients with nocturia do not have OAB. Most patients with

Table 8.2 Resolution of symptoms and incontinence reported from clinical trials of OAB medications in older people

Trial	Reduction in mean urgency episodes (v comparator, p)	Reduction in micturition frequency (v comparator, p)	Reduction in nocturia episodes (v comparator, p)	Reduction in incontinence episodes (v comparator, p)	Proportion with resolution of incontinence (v comparator, p)
Chapple (59) (12 weeks, darifenacin v placebo)	−88.6% v −77.9%, p = NS	−25.3% v −18.5%, p<0.01			70% v 58%, p = 0.021*
Malone-Lee (60) (12 weeks tolterodine v oxybutynin, pts over 50y)		−1.7 v −1.7, p = NS		= 1.3 (−54%) v −1.7 (−62%), (p not reported)	
Wagg (61) (12 weeks, solifenacin, pooled analysis v placebo)	−3.2 (5mg) −3.2 (10mg) v −1.1, p<0.05	−2.0 (5mg) −2.5 (10mg) v −1.1, p<0.05		−1.5 (5mg), −1.9 (10mg) v −1.0, p<0.005	49.1% (5mg), 47.3% (10mg) v 28.9%, p<0.001
Kraus (50) (pooled analysis, fesoterodine versus placebo >65-<75y and ≥75y v placebo)	>65-<75, −2.04 (4mg), −2.19 (8mg) v −0.77, p<0.05, ≥75, −1.13 (4mg), −2.01 (8mg) v −0.31, p<0.05 for 8mg	>65-<75, −1.83 (4mg), −1.68 (8mg) v −1.08, p<0.05, ≥75, −0.69 (4mg), −1.90 (8mg) v −0.36, p<0.05 for 4mg (>65) and 8mg (≥75)		>65-<75, −2.38 (4mg), −2.41 (8mg) v −0.98, p<0.05, ≥75, −1.87 (4mg), −2.44 (8mg) v −0.91, p<0.05 for 8mg	
Szonyi (62) (6 weeks oxybutynin combined with bladder retraining, results expressed as difference in change)	W = 577, (95% CI −27.0, −6.0), p = 0.0025		−6 (95% CI −5, 7)^ p = NS	−9.5 (95% CI −11.0,3.0)^ p = NS	

Table 8.2 (continued) Resolution of symptoms and incontinence reported from clinical trials of OAB medications in older people

Trial	Reduction in mean urgency episodes (v comparator, p)	Reduction in micturition frequency (v comparator, p)	Reduction in nocturia episodes (v comparator, p)	Reduction in incontinence episodes (v comparator, p)	Proportion with resolution of incontinence (v comparator, p)
Wagg (63) (12 week fesoterodine v placebo)	−3.47 v 1.92, p<0.001$	−1.91 v −0.93, p<0.001$	−1.0 v −0.7, p = 0.003$	−1.0 v −0.7, p = 0.729$	53% v 45%, p = 0.11**
Sand (64) (pooled analysis 12 weeks trospium v placebo)	−2.53 v −0.61, p = 0.004	−2.15 v −0.37, p<0.008	−0.76 v −0.08, p = 0.01	−1.77 v −0.54, p = 0.003	
DuBeau (65) (12 weeks, fesoterodine v placebo in older people identified as vulnerable on VES-13 scale)	−2.75 v −4.15, p = 0.001	−1.5 v −2.34, p≤0.001	−2.2 v −2.85, p = 0.002		36% v 50.8%, p = 0.002

*>50% reduction

^totalled over final 14 days and compared to first 14 days of run in

$change from baseline to week 12

**wet at baseline, dry at weeks 8 and 12

OAB do however have nocturia. Antimuscarinics are not usually efficacious for nocturia but they may be effective for nocturnal voids due to urgency. Other associated conditions include obstructive sleep apnoea, subclinical heart failure, loss of circadian variation in antidiuretic hormone levels, and other fluid-retaining states. Once a non–lower urinary tract underlying cause has been elucidated and, where possible, treated, nocturia may be classified as either nocturnal polyuria (>33% of total 24-hour urinary output overnight) or nocturnal frequency. Afternoon doses of loop diuretics (furosemide (74), bumetanide (75)) have some evidence supporting their use in nocturnal polyuria. The use of synthetic antidiuretic hormone (DDAVP) is also effective in reducing night-time urine output and increasing the mean amount of sleep (76–78). The drug is not licensed for use in people over the age of 65 years due to the risk of developing significant hyponatraemia, which occurs in up to 20% of adults within the first three days of treatment (79). However, if a baseline serum sodium is taken, followed by three days therapy and another estimation of serum sodium made (the patient having been instructed to stop their drug until notified otherwise), DDAVP may be used safely in selected people. Data suggest that serum sodium remains relatively stable for up to a year on therapy but it needs measuring should medication which might affect sodium balance (for example, antidepressants) be started or the patient develop an intercurrent illness (80).

7.6 **Surgery in older people**

There are data that support the use of anti-incontinence surgery in selected older people; there are no data on the frail elderly. Both botulinum toxin for urgency incontinence and midurethral tapes for stress urinary incontinence are effective (71–84). Hellberg et al. (85) showed that at three months, women ≥75 years old had a cure rate of 81.6% compared with a rate of 92.8% in women <75 years old. At later follow-up, regardless of duration since the tension-free vaginal tape (TVT) procedure, the proportion of women with cure for 'any' incontinence decreased with increasing age. In a randomized controlled trial of TVT versus six-month wait-list control, the intervention group at 6 months had a statistically significantly greater improvement in mean I-QOL score, patient satisfaction score, and urinary problem score (86). Older women do experience a greater number of adverse events than younger ones and the proportion reporting improvement/cure (however defined) may not be as high as in a younger group. There are fewer data, other than those for de-obstructing operative interventions, on surgery for incontinence in older men. Some case series for clam ileocystoplasty include men up to the age of 90, but they are undoubtedly carefully selected. Nevertheless, excellent operative outcomes for older people are achievable under the following conditions: appropriate selection and precautions; optimization of pre-morbid conditions; measures to reduce delirium; adequate hydration, nutrition, and analgesia; early proactive rehabilitation; treatment of postoperative delirium and functional impairment; and use of specialized care units. As with all surgery, due regard should be given to potential benefits and harms, and the potential patient appropriately counselled, taking note to include input from relevant caregivers where necessary.

7.7 Interventions for nocturnal enuresis

Night-time sleep in older people is often fragmented and disrupted. In care homes, much of this fragmentation and disruption is caused by noise, light, and care routines. When older people are dependent upon caregivers for going to bed, either in their own home or in a care facility, they may spend long periods of time in bed overnight—this in itself may predispose to enuresis.

Interventions that have been trialled in an attempt to enhance the quality and duration of sleep for residents with incontinence include daytime physical activity programmes either alone or combined with a night staff behaviour programme aimed at reducing noise, light, and sleep-disruptive care practices (87). Congestive heart failure, functional disability, depression, use of hypnotics, and nocturnal polyuria are all amenable to intervention in order to reduce the occurrence of enuresis.

8 Service delivery

Despite the plethora of national and international guidelines on treatment of incontinence, there remains little direction on how best to arrange services in order to deliver evidence-based care for older people. There is, unfortunately, a paucity of data on service models and delivery, and certainly much less on cost effectiveness. The seminal publication in the UK, *Good Practice in Continence Services* (88), was published in 2000; subsequent changes in organization of the Health Service in England and Wales have made this document obsolete although its principles remain sound. In 2010, the National Audit of Continence Care revealed that of the 55% (83/150) of continence services that declared themselves to be truly integrated, as defined by the standards in *Good Practice* only four truly were (89). A previous publication using data from the 2006 audit showed that the more integrated the service, the better the quality of care provided according to evidence-based standards (90). Following the publication of the National Institute for Health and Clinical Excellence (NICE) guidelines on incontinence in women, NICE produced guidance on commissioning a continence service aimed to deliver care compatible with its published guidance. Once again, however, the National Audits of Continence Care found that continence service provision was seldom a priority for commissioners of care. In fact, the delivery of continence care in England and Wales, at least for women, remains largely driven by specialists in hospitals (91). Continence services are an easy target for reduction in times of financial difficulty, hampering efforts to drive up standards. This is despite the fact that a large community survey across four European countries including the UK found that women preferred to be treated for UI by primary care providers, despite relatively free access to specialist services (92).

As far as trial evidence goes, there are some data from the UK and Australia about models of service which suggest that a community-delivered, nurse-led model can be effective, and that benefits to people can be maintained in the longer term (93, 94). These results were achieved despite the inherent instability of research conducted in the NHS environment. The Australian trials show that, regardless of the primary care model adopted, raising awareness and attention to the problem of continence results in higher standards of care delivery (95). Undoubtedly in many jurisdictions, remuneration drives practice. In England and Wales, repeated attempts at including a continence-related standard in the Quality Outcomes Framework have been unsuccessful. The societal balance of self-managed care/self-pay versus care provision has yet to be clarified in many health services. In the UK there is evidence of widespread rationing of continence-maintenance products in primary care, alongside inequitable assessments of eligibility for free provision (96)—a matter dear to the heart of many older people and their caregivers.

9 Conclusion

Urinary incontinence in older people constitutes a typical geriatric syndrome, and its original inclusion as one of the 'geriatric giants' was entirely rational. Incontinence in late life is often the result of many interacting contributory factors. Despite the relatively high prevalence of this condition in the elderly, the research evidence guiding effective management lags behind that for younger people. Services for older people often concentrate on control of the condition rather than active assessment and management. There is still much to do in this area; it is a field in which geriatricians should play an active role, but unfortunately there has been only a minority interest in this chronic medical condition from the profession. Salient summary points are shown in Box 8.1.

Box 8.1 Urinary incontinence

◆ Urinary incontinence in older people is a common condition with a marked impact on morbidity and quality of life of both people with the condition and their caregivers.

◆ There is probably no reason to assume that interventions which work in community-dwelling older people should not do so in the frail elderly.

◆ This assumption should guide practice when there is a dearth of direct evidence, but regard should be made to potential benefits, harm, and feasibility.

◆ Management involves a multicomponent intervention, common to those employed in other geriatric syndromes and an approach familiar to geriatricians.

Websites and key guidelines relevant to this chapter

European Urology Association guidelines on urinary incontinence—sets out guidance for management of both men and women:

<http://www.uroweb.org/gls/pdf/18_Urinary_Incontinence_LR.pdf>

NICE guidelines—national standards for management of urinary incontinence and prolapse in women (CG171) and lower urinary tract symptoms in men (CG97):

<http://guidance.nice.org.uk/CG171>

<http://www.nice.org.uk/nicemedia/live/12984/48557/48557.pdf>

References

1 Irwin DE, Milsom I, Hunskaar S, Reilly K, Kopp Z, Herschorn S, et al. Population-based survey of urinary incontinence, overactive bladder, and other lower urinary tract symptoms in five countries: results of the EPIC study. Eur Urol. 2006;50(6):1306–14; discussion 14–5.

2 Wakefield DB, Moscufo N, Guttmann CR, Kuchel GA, Kaplan RF, Pearlson G, et al. White matter hyperintensities predict functional decline in voiding, mobility, and cognition in older adults. J Am Geriatr Soc. 2010;58(2):275–81.

3 Milsom I, Abrams P, Cardozo L, Roberts RG, Thuroff J, Wein AJ. How widespread are the symptoms of an overactive bladder and how are they managed? A population-based prevalence study. BJU Int. 2001;87(9):760–6.

4 Wennberg AL, Molander U, Fall M, Edlund C, Peeker R, Milsom I. A longitudinal population-based survey of urinary incontinence, overactive bladder, and other lower urinary tract symptoms in women. Eur Urol. 2009 Apr;55(4):783–91.

5 Malmsten UG, Molander U, Peeker R, Irwin DE, Milsom I. Urinary incontinence, overactive bladder, and other lower urinary tract symptoms: a longitudinal population-based survey in men aged 45–103 years. Eur Urol. 2010;**58**(1):149–56.

6 van Melick HH, van Venrooij GE, Eckhardt MD, Boon TA. A randomized controlled trial comparing transurethral resection of the prostate, contact laser prostatectomy and electrovaporization in men with benign prostatic hyperplasia: analysis of subjective changes, morbidity and mortality. J Urol. 2003;**169**(4):1411–6.

7 Goluboff ET, Saidi JA, Mazer S, Bagiella E, Heitjan DF, Benson MC, et al. Urinary continence after radical prostatectomy: the Columbia experience. J Urol. 1998;**159**(4): 1276–80.

8 Moinzadeh A, Shunaigat AN, Libertino JA. Urinary incontinence after radical retropubic prostatectomy: the outcome of a surgical technique. BJU Int. 2003;**92**(4):355–9.

9 Shaw C, Gupta RD, Bushnell DM, Assassa RP, Abrams P, Wagg A, et al. The extent and severity of urinary incontinence amongst women in UK GP waiting rooms. Fam Pract. 2006;**23**(5):497–506.

10 Khullar V, Cardozo L, Dmochowski R. Mixed incontinence: current evidence and future perspectives. Neurourol Urodyn. 2010;**29**(4):618–22.

11 Burgio KL, Locher JL, Ives DG, Hardin JM, Newman AB, Kuller LH. Nocturnal enuresis in community-dwelling older adults. J Am Geriatr Soc. 1996;**44**(2):139–43.

12 Sakamoto K, Blaivas JG. Adult onset nocturnal enuresis. J Urol. 2001;**165**(6 Pt 1): 1914–7.

13 Bonde HV, Sejr T, Erdmann L, Meyhoff HH, Lendorf A, Rosenkilde P, et al. Residual urine in 75-year-old men and women. A normative population study. Scand J Urol Nephrol. 1996;**30**(2):89–91.

14 Kolman C, Girman CJ, Jacobsen SJ, Lieber MM. Distribution of post-void residual urine volume in randomly selected men. J Urol. 1999;**161**(1):122–7.

15 Huang AJ, Brown JS, Boyko EJ, Moore EE, Scholes D, Walter LC, et al. Clinical significance of postvoid residual volume in older ambulatory women. J Am Geriatr Soc. 2011;**59**(8):1452–8.

16 Malone-Lee J, Wahedna, I. Characterisation of detrusor contractile function in relation to old-age. Br J Urol. 1993;**72**:873–80.

17 Susset JG, Servot-Viguier D, Lamy F, Madernas P, Black R. Collagen in 155 human bladders. Invest Urol. 1978;**16**(3):204–6.

18 Mitchell JP. Management of chronic urinary retention. Brit Med J. 1984;**289**(6444): 515–6.

19 Brown JS, Vittinghoff E, Wyman JF, Stone KL, Nevitt MC, Ensrud KE, et al. Urinary incontinence: does it increase risk for falls and fractures? Study of Osteoporotic Fractures Research Group. J Am Geriatr Soc. 2000;**48**(7):721–5.

20 Thom DH, Haan MN, Van Den Eeden SK. Medically recognized urinary incontinence and risks of hospitalization, nursing home admission and mortality. Age Ageing. 1997;**26**(5):367–74.

21 Zorn BH, Montgomery H, Pieper K, Gray M, Steers WD. Urinary incontinence and depression. J Urol. 1999;**162**(1):82–4.

22 Cigolle CT, Langa KM, Kabeto MU, Tian Z, Blaum CS. Geriatric conditions and disability: the Health and Retirement Study. Ann Intern Med. 2007;**147**(3):156–64.

23 Smith AL, Wang P-C, Anger JT, Mangione CM, Trejo L, Rodriguez LV, et al. Correlates of urinary incontinence in community-dwelling older Latinos. J Am Geriatr Soc. 2010;**58**:1170–6.

24 Barentsen JA, Visser E, Hofstetter H, Maris AM, Dekker JH, de Bock GH. Severity, not type, is the main predictor of decreased quality of life in elderly women with urinary incontinence: a population-based study as part of a randomized controlled trial in primary care. Health Qual Life Outcomes. 2012;10:153.

25 Khatutsky G, Walsh EG, Brown DW. Urinary incontinence, functional status, and health-related quality of life among Medicare beneficiaries enrolled in the program for all-inclusive care for the elderly and dual eligible demonstration special needs plans. J Ambul Care Manage. 2013;**36**(1):35–49.

26 Ko Y, Lin SJ, Salmon JW, Bron MS. The impact of urinary incontinence on quality of life of the elderly. Am J Manag Care. 2005;**11**(4 Suppl):S103–11.

27 Coyne KS, Sexton CC, Irwin DE, Kopp ZS, Kelleher CJ, Milsom I. The impact of overactive bladder, incontinence and other lower urinary tract symptoms on quality of life, work productivity, sexuality and emotional well-being in men and women: results from the EPIC study. BJU Int. 2008;**101**(11):1388–95.

28 Gotoh M, Matsukawa Y, Yoshikawa Y, Funahashi Y, Kato M, Hattori R. Impact of urinary incontinence on the psychological burden of family caregivers. Neurourol Urodyn. 2009;**28**(6):492–6.

29 Irwin DE, Mungapen L, Milsom I, Kopp Z, Reeves P, Kelleher C. The economic impact of overactive bladder syndrome in six Western countries. BJU Int. 2009;**103**(2):202–9.

30 McMurdo ME, Roberts H, Parker S, Wyatt N, May H, Goodman C, et al. Improving recruitment of older people to research through good practice. Age Ageing. 2011;**40**(6):659–65.

31 Wagg A, Gibson W, Johnson T 3rd, Markland A, Palmer MH, Kuchel G, Szonyi G, Kirschner-Hermanns R. Urinary incontinence in frail elderly persons: report from the 5th International Consultation on Incontinence. Neurourol Urodyn. doi: 10.1002/nau.22602. Epub ahead of print 2014 Apr 2. PMID: 24700771

32 Landefeld CS, Bowers BJ, Feld AD, Hartmann KE, Hoffman E, Ingber MJ, et al. National Institutes of Health state-of-the-science conference statement: prevention of fecal and urinary incontinence in adults. Ann Intern Med. 2008;**148**(6):449–58.

33 Roe B, Ostaszkiewicz J, Milne J, Wallace S. Systematic reviews of bladder training and voiding programmes in adults: a synopsis of findings from data analysis and outcomes using metastudy techniques. J Adv Nurs. 2007;**57**(1):15–31.

34 Palmer MH. Effectiveness of prompted voiding for incontinent nursing home residents. In: BM Melnyk, E Fineout-Overholt, eds. Evidence-based practice in nursing and healthcare: A guide to best practice. Philadelphia: Lippincott Williams & Wilkins; 2005. p. 20–30.

35 Palmer MH. Use of health behavior change theories to guide urinary incontinence research. Nurs Res. 2004;**53**(6 Suppl):S49–55.

36 Roe B, Milne J, Ostaszkiewicz J, Wallace S. Systematic reviews of bladder training and voiding programmes in adults: a synopsis of findings on theory and methods using metastudy techniques. J Adv Nurs. 2007;**57**(1):3–14.

37 Ostaszkiewicz J, Johnston L, Roe B. Timed voiding for the management of urinary incontinence in adults. J Urol. 2005;**173**(4):1262–3.

38 Schnelle JF, MacRae PG, Ouslander JG, Simmons SF, Nitta M. Functional Incidental Training, mobility performance, and incontinence care with nursing home residents. J Am Geriatr Soc. 1995;43(12):1356–62.

39 Ouslander JG, Griffiths P, McConnell E, Riolo L, Schnelle J. Functional Incidental Training: applicability and feasibility in the Veterans Affairs nursing home patient population. J Am Med Dir Assoc. 2005;6(2):121–7.

40 Bates-Jensen BM, Alessi CA, Al-Samarrai NR, Schnelle JF. The effects of an exercise and incontinence intervention on skin health outcomes in nursing home residents. J Am Geriatr Soc. 2003;51(3):348–55.

41 Jirovec MM. The impact of daily exercise on the mobility, balance and urine control of cognitively impaired nursing home residents. Int J Nurs Stud. 1991;28(2):145–51.

42 van Houten P, Achterberg W, Ribbe M. Urinary incontinence in disabled elderly women: a randomized clinical trial on the effect of training mobility and toileting skills to achieve independent toileting. Gerontology. 2007;53(4):205–10.

43 Sugaya K, Nishijima S, Owan T, Oda M, Miyazato M, Ogawa Y. Effects of walking exercise on nocturia in the elderly. Biomed Res. 2007;28(2):101–5.

44 Booth J, Kumlien S, Zang Y. Promoting urinary continence with older people: key issues for nurses. Int J Older People Nurs. 2009;4(1):63–9.

45 Dingwall L. Promoting effective continence care for older people: a literature review. Br J Nurs. 2008;17(3):166–72.

46 Wright J, McCormack B, Coffey A, McCarthy G. Evaluating the context within which continence care is provided in rehabilitation units for older people. Int J Older People Nurs. 2007;2(1):9–19.

47 Vinsnes AG, Harkless GE, Nyronning S. Unit-based intervention to improve urinary incontinence in frail elderly. Nordic J Nurs Res Clin Stud. 2007;27(3):53.

48 Diokno AC, Sampselle CM, Herzog AR, Raghunathan TE, Hines S, Messer KL, et al. Prevention of urinary incontinence by behavioral modification program: a randomized, controlled trial among older women in the community. J Urol. 2004;171(3):1165–71.

49 Choo MS, Song C, Kim JH, Choi JB, Lee JY, Chung BS, et al. Changes in overactive bladder symptoms after discontinuation of successful 3-month treatment with an antimuscarinic agent: a prospective trial. J Urol. 2005;174(1):201–4.

50 Kraus SR, Ruiz-Cerda JL, Martire D, Wang JT, Wagg AS. Efficacy and tolerability of fesoterodine in older and younger subjects with overactive bladder. Urology. 2010;76:1350–7.

51 Wagg A, Wyndaele JJ, Sieber P. Efficacy and tolerability of solifenacin in elderly subjects with overactive bladder syndrome: a pooled analysis. Am J Geriatr Pharmacother. 2006;4(1):14–24.

52 Wagg A, Compion G, Fahey A, Siddiqui E. Persistence with prescribed antimuscarinic therapy for overactive bladder: a UK experience. BJU Int. 2012 Dec;110(11):1767–74. doi: 10.1111/j.1464-410X.2012.11023.x. Epub 2012 Mar 12.

53 Lackner T, Wyman J, McCarthy T, Monigold M, Davey C. Randomized, placebo-controlled trial of the cognitive effect, safety, and tolerability of oral extended-release oxybutynin in cognitively impaired nursing home residents with urge urinary incontinence. J Am Geriatr Soc. 2008;56:862–70.

54 Sand P, et al. Oxybutynin transdermal system improves the quality of life in adults with overactive bladder: a multi-centre community based, randomized study. BJU Int. 2007;**99**:836–44.

55 DuBeau CE, Ouslander JG, Johnson TM, Wyman JF, Kraus SR, Griebling TL, Newman DK, Sun F, Catuogno J, Bavendam T. Fesoterodine is effective and well tolerated in vulnerable elderly subjects with urgency incontinence: A double-blind, placebo-controlled study. Atlanta: American Urological Association; 2012.

56 Buser N, Ivic S, Kessler TM, Kessels AG, Bachmann LM. Efficacy and adverse events of antimuscarinics for treating overactive bladder: network meta-analyses. Eur Urol. 2012 Dec;**62**(6):1040–60. doi: 10.1016/j.eururo.2012.08.060. Epub 2012 Sep 7.

57 Gomes T, Juurlink DN, Ho JM, Schneeweiss S, Mamdani MM. Risk of serious falls associated with oxybutynin and tolterodine: a population based study. J Urol. 2011; **186**(4):1340–4.

58 Lackner TE, Wyman JF, McCarthy TC, Monigold M, Davey C. Efficacy of oral extended-release oxybutynin in cognitively impaired older nursing home residents with urge urinary incontinence: a randomized placebo-controlled trial. J Amer Med Dir Assoc. 2011;**12**:639–47.

59 Chapple C, DuBeau C, Ebinger U, Rekeda L, Viegas A. Darifenacin treatment of patients >or = 65 years with overactive bladder: results of a randomized, controlled, 12-week trial. Curr Med Res Opin. 2007;**23**(10):2347–58.

60 Malone-Lee J, Shaffu B, Anand C, Powell C. Tolterodine: superior tolerability than and comparable efficacy to oxybutynin in individuals 50 years old or older with overactive bladder: a randomized controlled trial. J Urol. 2001;**165**(5):1452–6.

61 Wagg A, Wyndaele JJ, Sieber P. Efficacy and tolerability of solifenacin in elderly subjects with overactive bladder syndrome: a pooled analysis. Am J Geriatr Pharmacother. 2006;**4**(1):14–24.

62 Szonyi G, Collas DM, Ding YY, Malone-Lee JG. Oxybutynin with bladder retraining for detrusor instability in elderly people: a randomized controlled trial. Age Ageing. 1995;**24**(4):287–91.

63 Wagg A, Khullar V, Marscall-Kehrel D, Michel M, Oelke M, Tincello D, Darekar A, Ebel Bitoun C, Osterloh I, Weinstein D. Assessment of fesoterodine treatment in older people with overactive bladder: results of SOFIA, a double blind, placebo controlled pan-European trial. Proc Meet Eur Urol Assoc. 2010;**880**.

64 Sand PK, Johnson Ii TM, Rovner ES, Ellsworth PI, Oefelein MG, Staskin DR. Trospium chloride once-daily extended release is efficacious and tolerated in elderly subjects (aged >/= 75 years) with overactive bladder syndrome. BJU Int. 2011;**107**(4): 612–20.

65 DuBeau CE, Kraus SR, Griebling TL, Newman DK, Wyman JF, Johnson TM 2nd, Ouslander JG, Sun F, Gong J, Bavendam T. Effect of fesoterodine in vulnerable elderly subjects with urgency incontinence: a double-blind, placebo-controlled trial. J Urol. 2014 Feb;**191**(2):395–404. doi: 10.1016/j.juro.2013.08.027. Epub 2013 Aug 21.

66 Wagg A, Cardozo L, Nitti VW, Castro-Diaz D, Auerbach S, Blauwet MB, Siddiqui E. The efficacy and tolerability of the β3-adrenoceptor agonist mirabegron for the treatment of symptoms of overactive bladder in older patients.Age Ageing. Epub ahead of print 2014 Mar 14. PMID: 24610862

67 Kay GG, Maruff P, Scholfield D, Malhotra B, Whelan L, Darekar A, et al. Evaluation of cognitive function in healthy older subjects treated with fesoterodine. Postgrad Med. 2012;**124**(3):7–15.

68 Kay GG, Staskin DR, Macdiarmid S, McIlwain M, Dahl NV. Cognitive effects of oxybutynin chloride topical gel in older healthy subjects: a 1-week, randomized, double-blind, placebo- and active-controlled study. Clin Drug Invest. 2012;**32**(10):707–14.

69 Lipton RB, Kolodner K, Wesnes K. Assessment of cognitive function of the elderly population: effects of darifenacin. J Urol. 2005;**173**(2):493–8.

70 Staskin D, Kay G, Tannenbaum C, Goldman HB, Bhashi K, Ling J, Oefelein MG. Trospium chloride has no effect on memory testing and is assay undetectable in the central nervous system of older patients with overactive bladder. Int J Clin Pract. 2010;**64**(9):1294–300.

71 Wagg A. The cognitive burden of anticholinergics in the elderly- implications for the treatment of overactive bladder. Eur Urol Rev. 2012;**7**(1):42–9.

72 Wagg A, Dale M, Compion G, Stow B Tretter R. Solifenacin and cognitive impairment in elderly people with mild cognitive impairment: the SENIOR study. Eur Urol. 2013 Jul;**64**(1):74–81. doi: 10.1016/j.eururo.2013.01.002. Epub 1013 Jan 11.

73 Wesnes KA, Edgar C, Tretter RN, Bolodeoku J. Exploratory pilot study assessing the risk of cognitive impairment or sedation in the elderly following single doses of solifenacin 10 mg. Expert Opin Drug Safety. 2009;**8**(6):615–26.

74 Reynard JM, Cannon A, Yang Q, Abrams P. A novel therapy for nocturnal polyuria: a double-blind randomized trial of frusemide against placebo. Br J Urol. 1998;**81**(2): 215–8.

75 Pedersen PA, Johansen PB. Prophylactic treatment of adult nocturia with bumetanide. Br J Urol. 1988;**62**(2):145–7.

76 Asplund R, Sundberg, B, Bergtsson, P. Oral desmopressin for nocturnal polyuria in elderly subjects: a double blind, placebo-controlled randomized exploratory study. BJU Int. 1999;**83**:591–5.

77 Asplund R, Sundberg B, Bengtsson P. Oral desmopressin for nocturnal polyuria in elderly subjects: a double-blind, placebo-controlled randomized exploratory study. BJU Int. 1999;**83**(6):591–5.

78 Rezakhaniha B, Arianpour N, Siroosbakhat S. Efficacy of desmopressin in treatment of nocturia in elderly men. J Res Med Sci. 2011;**16**(4):516–23.

79 Weatherall M. The risk of hyponatremia in older adults using desmopressin for nocturia: a systematic review and meta-analysis. Neurourol Urodyn. 2004;**23**(4):302–5.

80 Cornu JN, Abrams P, Chapple CR, Dmochowski RR, Lemack GE, Michel MC, et al. A contemporary assessment of nocturia: definition, epidemiology, pathophysiology, and management: a systematic review and meta-analysis. Eur Urol. 2012 Nov;**62**(5):877–90. doi: 10.1016/j.eururo.2013.01.002. Epub 2012 Jul 20.

81 Karantanis E, Fynes MM, Stanton SL. The tension-free vaginal tape in older women. BJOG: Int J Obstet Gynaecol. 2004;**111**:837–41.

82 Lo TS, Huang HJ, Chang CL, Wong SY, Horng SG, Liang CC. Use of intravenous anesthesia for tension-free vaginal tape therapy in elderly women with genuine stress incontinence. Urology. 2002;**59**(3):349–53.

83 Sevestre S, Ciofu C, Deval B, Traxer O, Amarenco G, Haab F. Results of the tension-free vaginal tape technique in the elderly. Eur Urol. 2003;**44**(1):128–31.

84 White WM, Pickens RB, Doggweiler R, Klein FA. Short-term efficacy of botulinum toxin a for refractory overactive bladder in the elderly population. J Urol. 2008;**180**(6):2522–6.

85 Hellberg D, Holmgren C, Lanner L, Nilsson S. The very obese woman and the very old woman: tension free vaginal tape for the treatment of stress urinary incontinence. Int Urogynaecol J Pelvic Floor Dysfunct. 2007;**18**(4):423–9.

86 Campeau L, Tu LM, Lemieux MC, Naud A, Karsenty G, Schick E, et al. A multicenter, prospective, randomized clinical trial comparing tension-free vaginal tape surgery and no treatment for the management of stress urinary incontinence in elderly women. Neurourol Urodyn. 2007;**26**(7):990–4.

87 Alessi CA, Yoon EJ, Schnelle JF, Al-Samarrai NR, Cruise PA. A randomized trial of a combined physical activity and environmental intervention in nursing home residents: do sleep and agitation improve? J Am Geriatr Soc. 1999;**47**(7):784–91.

88 Good Practice in Continence Services. Department of Health London: HMSO; 2000.

89 Wagg A. National Audit of Continence Care. London: Royal College of Physicians of London; 2010.

90 Wagg A, Lowe D, Peel P, Potter J. Do self-reported 'integrated' continence services provide high-quality continence care? Age Ageing. 2009;**38**(6):730–3.

91 Wagg A, Duckett J, McClurg D, Harari D, Lowe D. To what extent are national guidelines for the management of urinary incontinence in women adhered? Data from a national audit. BJOG: Int J Obstet Gynaecol. 2011;**118**(13):1592–1600.

92 O'Donnell M, Viktrup L, Hunskaar S. The role of general practitioners in the initial management of women with urinary incontinence in France, Germany, Spain and the UK. Eur J Gen Pract. 2007;**13**(1):20–6.

93 Williams KS, Assassa RP, Cooper NJ, Turner DA, Shaw C, Abrams KR, et al. Clinical and cost-effectiveness of a new nurse-led continence service: a randomised controlled trial. Br J Gen Pract. 2005;**55**(518):696–703.

94 Williams KS, Assassa RP, Gillies CL, Abrams KR, Turner DA, Shaw C, et al. A randomized controlled trial of the effectiveness of pelvic floor therapies for urodynamic stress and mixed incontinence. BJU Int. 2006;**98**(5):1043–50.

95 Byles JE, Chiarelli P, Hacker AH, Bruin C, Cockburn J, Parkinson L. An evaluation of three community-based projects to improve care for incontinence. Int Urogynecol J Pelvic Floor Dysfunct. 2005;**16**(1):29–38 [discussion].

96 Desai N, Keane, T, Wagg, A, Wardle, J. Provision of continence pads by the continence services in Great Britain: fair all round? J Wound Ostomy Continence Nurs. 2008;**35**(5): 510–4.

Chapter 9

Depressions in later life: heterogeneity and co-morbidities

David Anderson

Key points

- Depression in older people is among the most disabling of conditions.
- Depression is the most common and treatable mental disorder in later life.
- Depression in older people is undertreated in absolute terms and compared to younger adults.
- Depression is a heterogeneous disorder: objectively defining sub-types will be essential to developing more specific treatments.

---

1 Introduction

Depression is a term that means many things to many people. Consequently, any discourse could be criticized for being non-specific and over inclusive, or too specific and exclusive. Therein lie many of the difficulties of understanding and discussing the subject. Colloquial use describing a normal emotion of sadness is different from medical diagnostics, though there is dispute about diagnostic criteria, the arbitrary threshold when normal becomes pathological, and whether current diagnostic criteria are discriminating (1). As a clinical syndrome, diagnosis depends entirely on the clinician's interpretation of symptoms.

Classifications give the impression of a single condition rated mild to severe by cumulative symptom score. Yet, depression is clearly a heterogeneous group of disorders with overlapping core features of anhedonia, fatigue, loss of interest, and low mood. It may occur with biological symptoms (appetite, weight, sleep), with psychotic symptoms (delusions, hallucinations), with motor symptoms (retardation, agitation); as variants like psychotic, melancholic, bipolar, brief, organic, major, and minor; with severity from mild to severe; and as a single episode or recurrent.

Medical co-morbidities, typical of older people, complicate matters further, because it is often difficult to know whether symptoms, particularly biological ones, should be attributed to depression or the physical condition. In a study of medical admissions over age 70, fine changes to the application of diagnostic criteria—removing biological symptoms and substituting psychological symptoms—reduced the prevalence from 20.7% to 15% (2).

Nevertheless, a condition that can cause profound loss of function and capability, associated with mood change, physical symptoms, impaired intellectual function, and altered thought and perception has been recognized since the time of Hippocrates and Galen. The condition was described vividly in the mid-nineteenth century by Esquirol (3), who reported how patients succumbed to malnutrition and infection; it was first captured in the English language by Robert Burton's autobiographical account of melancholia (4).

2 Incidence and impact

Depression is among the most disabling of conditions. In 2008 (5) it was declared the third highest global cause of loss of disability-adjusted life years, the highest in middle- and high-income countries, and projected to be the highest globally by 2030. Depression is associated with a decrement in health greater than common chronic diseases (6). Further, it complicates the treatment of other medical conditions by virtue of apathy, loss of engagement, non-compliance, and secondary physical disability. As a risk factor for coronary heart disease, depression is reported to be as significant as diabetes and smoking (7). There is evidence that depression is also a risk factor for stroke, colorectal cancer, back pain, irritable bowel syndrome, multiple sclerosis, and possibly type II diabetes (8). Untreated depression in older people approximately doubles mortality rate (9). Depression accounts for over 80% of deaths by suicide of older people (10). Deliberate self-harm in older people usually represents a failed suicide attempt (very different from younger people when mental illness is rarely implicated and self-harm is impulsive) and the recognized determinants of suicide are evident (11). The risk of suicide after deliberate self-harm increases markedly with age (12), especially if there has been a previous episode (13). A prospective study of self-harm in adults over age 60 found the risk of suicide was 67 times higher than the general population in the following 12 months, with men over age 75 at highest risk (14).

3 **Depression in the older person**

The symptoms of depression in later life appear similar to younger age groups (although, it is true, older people manifest more somatic symptoms and more agitation, experience less guilt and less reduction of sexual libido, and their symptoms tend to be more severe) (15). Nevertheless, we cannot assume, without question, that depression is the same for both age groups. Indeed, a criticism of approaches to late-onset depression would be the extrapolation of an evidence base from research with younger populations. The trend in classifications and some interpretations of equality that disregard age as a variable should not make us complacent in believing that late-onset disorders can be understood and approached in the same way as those of younger people. To do so may be indirect age discrimination (16) and, even if symptoms are similar, a very different psychosocial context and co-morbidity alters management (Box 9.1).

There are substantially fewer studies of depression in later life and, it could be argued, the treatment evidence base for an older population with multiple co-morbidities barely exists (other than at the level of clinical experience), because people with co-morbidities on multiple drug treatments are usually excluded from clinical trials. One could also argue that this is when specialists, working with a familiar set of circumstances, become important.

Box 9.1 **Characteristics of depression in older people compared to younger adults**

- symptoms—more somatic, agitation, and cognitive impairment
  - less guilt and less loss of sexual libido
  - tending to more severe
- higher suicidality and greater risk of suicide after deliberate self-harm
- vascular brain changes more common
- more often complicated by multimorbidity
- longer duration of maintenance treatment to prevent relapse
- greater sensitivity to adverse effects of antidepressants
- less often diagnosed or referred to psychiatry
- less research done on older people
- less quality guidance available.

4 **Epidemiology and causes**

The EURODEP collaboration found the prevalence of case-level depression—that is, depression suitable for intervention—varied from 8.8% to 23.6% using the same standardized diagnostic tool in community studies of people over age 65 years in Europe (17). A systematic review of all community studies reported prevalence of 0.4–35% with an average of 13.5% (1.8% severe) in those over age 55 (18).

Explanations of these variations elude us, though there is broad agreement that being widowed or divorced, having low educational attainment, poor self-rated health, functional and cognitive impairment, poor social networks, and socio-economic adversity all increase the likelihood of depression. Protective factors include good physical health, a confidante, marriage for males, a strong social network, and religious faith. Genetics probably play a part, though not by single-gene effects, and probably less so for late-onset depression; further, genetic effects are likely to vary by subtype.

By virtue of an ageing population it is predicted that the number of people in England over age 75 with depression will increase by 30% from 2008–2026. For those over 85, the number jumps to 80% (19).

The amine hypothesis of depression (20) was a milestone in the history of psychiatry, providing both a biological explanation and the scientific basis for drug treatment. Further understanding came from recognizing the social determinants of adversity and life events (21), cognitive theories of depression (22), and the relationship with physical illness, disability, and handicap (23). More recently, vascular depression describes a sub-group of late-onset cases associated with extensive ischaemic changes (particularly frontal and basal ganglia) found on brain magnetic resonance imaging (24).

That all of these provide credible frameworks for understanding and treating depression in different people attests to the heterogeneity of this condition.

4.1 **Treatment and outcome**

Depression can be self-limiting. More than 100 years ago, and before antidepressant treatments, the father of modern psychiatry, Emil Kraepelin (25), noted that one third of patients with melancholia made a complete recovery (these were severe or psychotic asylum cases). Due to the seriousness of suicidal thinking, Kraepelin thought all needed treatment in the asylum. In the seminal study into the mental disorders of late life, Roth (26) provided elegantly descriptive evidence that these were not all variants of senile dementia. Rather, depression differed from the others: patients with depression showed the ability to recover and be discharged from the asylum. Roth reported that 33% of depressed patients admitted in 1934 or 1936 (before treatment) were discharged within six months, whereas the rate climbed to 58% in 1948 and 1949 after introduction of electroconvulsive therapy (ECT), the first antidepressant treatment.

More recently, a community study of essentially untreated depressed elders found 22% of those completing five-year follow-up were recovered (27). A longitudinal primary-care study of people over age 55 found that the median duration of a major depressive episode was 18 months. Although no more than 40% of the patients received treatment, 35%, 60%, and 68% recovered at one, two, and three years, respectively (28).

Treating depression in later life follows the same principles as for younger people. Antidepressants and psychological approaches are equally as effective for older people (29, 30). Antidepressant monotherapy response is 50–60%; number needed to treat ranges from four to eight depending on antidepressant class, but the majority of antidepressant trials with older people exclude those with physical illness (29). Debate continues about the superiority of one antidepressant class over another and there is currently no reliable way to predict who will respond to which treatment (31). Choice of antidepressant is often determined by side-effect profile, which varies by class; all present risks with older people (32). Detailed discussion of these differences is beyond the scope of this chapter.

Sertraline and citalopram have, possibly, the best risk-benefit ratio (33) and are least likely to affect the p450 enzyme system and interact with other medications. A caveat is that citalopram causes dose-related prolongation of the QTc interval (34). An early response predicts the best recovery (35). Response to ECT is at least as good for older people who show an improvement in cognitive function proportionately greater than younger subjects (36, 37). A systematic review suggests that 52% who fail to respond to a single antidepressant will respond to alternative pharmacotherapy, though the authors note the paucity of good quality studies and an absence of guidance in comparison to younger adults (38). The time involved working through these alternatives can be frustrating and disheartening for patients.

Psychological treatments should be used for mild depression but the best outcome for moderate and severe depression is achieved by combining psychological and pharmacological treatments (39). Following recovery, antidepressants need to be continued longer with older people; active treatment confers benefit over placebo up to 21 months with two and half times reduction of relapse rate (40). Up to 90% of those maintained on placebo have recurrence within three years but with prophylaxis this is more than halved (41). It is a remitting and relapsing illness for most.

Despite this, depression in later life is far less likely to be treated than in younger adults. Not all older people discuss depression with their physician. Instead, most attend primary care with physical complaints, and some studies find that the diagnosis is often missed in primary care. Even when recognized, depression in the older person is less likely to be treated or managed by referral to psychiatry services (42, 43). It is estimated that around one in six older depressed people in the UK receive treatment of any sort. Whereas 50% of depressed younger adults are referred to psychiatry services, the rate is only 6% for older people (44). So, for every 1 million depressed older people, 850,000 receive no treatment—approximately 2.5 million nationwide. That 4% of the depressed in a community study of older people were in receipt of antidepressants while 80% were receiving prescriptions for other medical conditions (45) suggests that depression prompts less of a response from clinicians than physical conditions.

That adversity and illness become common in later life may tempt clinicians to conclude that depression is a natural reaction not needing treatment. Such stereotypical perception that depression is just a consequence of old age is not upheld by community studies (46). The old distinction between reactive and endogenous depressions, implying the former was natural and the latter in need of treatment, was dispelled once it was shown that both respond equally to treatment. Aetiology informs the type of treatment, not its need, just as the cause of pain informs the method, not the need of pain relief.

While the best quality evidence for treatment is physical and structured psychological (e.g. cognitive behaviour therapy) approaches that minimize disability, promotion of independence, supportive therapies, and social networks will be an important part of a treatment plan for many. Systematic review suggests that tailored structured exercise may reduce depression severity in older people (47).

5 Co-morbidities and curiosities

In a general hospital, the prevalence of depression is approximately double that in the community and higher with most long-term conditions. The mean number of common conditions affecting depressed people over age 65 in the UK is 4.9 (48). Here, physical symptoms and context make diagnosis more difficult. Focusing on non-physical symptoms improves diagnostic specificity for severe and persistent depressions (2).

Pooled data from controlled trials with a range of co-morbidities show that antidepressants are effective, though not always well tolerated (49). Studies reveal interesting differences with different co-morbidities that might point to differences in pathogenesis and some particular effects of antidepressants. For example, 35% of people with Parkinson's disease (PD) have prevalent clinically relevant depressive symptoms (50), but depression is not clearly related to severity of motor symptoms or physical disability (51). In the context of this bradykinetic condition, it is interesting to consider a view that melancholia (a biological depressive concept) is characterized by psychomotor retardation and not mood symptoms (52), that psychomotor retardation is a predictor of response to ECT (53, 54), and that observational studies find improvement in motor symptoms from ECT in the absence of depression (55). Psychomotor slowing is the hallmark of subcortical diseases. The best treatment evidence to date is probably for tricyclic antidepressants when the comparator, a selective serotonin reuptake inhibitor (SSRI), was no better than placebo (56). Anecdotally, PD specialists have treated depression with amitriptyline at low doses. Is the anticholinergic effect important? Amitriptyline is rarely used now to treat depression in general but used widely to control neuropathic pain (57). Pramipexole, a dopa agonist, may have antidepressant properties (58). So, are these depressions or manifestations of PD?

Large studies of post–myocardial infarction and unstable angina confirm the safety and benefit of new-generation antidepressants when the tricyclic group is cardiotoxic (59, 60). Subsequent incidence of fatal and non-fatal myocardial ischaemia is lower in those treated with SSRIs (61), attributed to reduced coagulation from inhibition of serotonin reuptake by platelets, which is not found with tricyclic antidepressants (62). Reduced coagulation is also the reason SSRIs may cause increased risk of bleeding.

Antidepressants are effective for treatment of depression after stroke (63). SSRIs may improve frontal executive function regardless of any antidepressant effect (64). Frontal dysexecutive syndrome predicts antidepressant resistance (41), as does vascular depression. It may be that treatment of vascular depression focuses on influencing its presumed vascular basis, and there is preliminary interest in the use of calcium channel blockers (65). Cerebrovascular disease is the most likely explanation for persisting cognitive deficits with depression in older age (66).

Persuading older people with COPD to take antidepressant drugs has been strikingly unsuccessful and emphasis has shifted from antidepressants to a problem-based treatment intervention (67). The best evidence for treatment of depression in COPD and chronic heart failure is for cardiorespiratory rehabilitation taking a holistic, educational, and problem-based approach (8).

New-generation antidepressants are disappointingly ineffective in people with Alzheimer's disease (68), yet depression appears to be a risk factor for developing dementia (69, 70). As antidepressants and mood stabilizers seem to increase hippocampal neurogenesis, will they have a new role in the future?

So there is a constant problem of heterogeneity since no single treatment is sufficient, and it seems unlikely that these depressions are all the same condition. Unravelling this is critical to making treatment more specific. Comorbidity, treatment tolerance, and polypharmacy make treatment of the older person more complicated.

6 Future developments

It will be our ability to disentangle this heterogeneity and recognize specific disorders defined by objective diagnostic criteria that will advance our knowledge of the pathophysiology of depression and lead to disorder-specific treatments. Historically, physical medicine has confronted the same challenge. Unless mental disorder has nothing in common with physical disorder, then psychiatry will need to progress along this path. Novel antidepressants continue to be developed, but even though they may be better tolerated, randomized controlled trials of a heterogeneous disorder will continue to produce the same varied and contentious results.

In the meantime, early detection and treatment of depression has the best prognosis. Care management reduces mortality with older depressed people (71), and antidepressants and lithium salts reduce suicides (72, 73). Better physical health and greater prevention of disability and handicap from long-term conditions should reduce incidence. The recognition that brain white-matter lesions may be an important aetiological factor in late-life depression (74) and that blood pressure control reduces progression of such lesions (75, 76) means the management of vascular risk may have similar benefit. There is mutual gain for closer collaboration between psychiatry and medicine. Reducing social inequalities and socio-economic adversity lies with politicians.

7 Conclusion

Depression is a clinical syndrome, the most common mental health problem in later life, with numbers increasing as populations age. It is the most treatable mental disorder, yet undertreated. There is concern that the pre-eminence of dementia on the age-related health agenda could leave depression in later life overlooked, even though depression is two to three times more common. It deserves a more prominent position on the health agenda and within that agenda there has to be greater focus on research and service delivery for older people and those with complex co-morbidities (77).

In the 1960s and 1970s, biological and psychosocial hypotheses for the origins of depression gave us a scientific rationale for the development of evidence-based treatments. Since then progress has been slow, although treatment has become more refined and safer. Our understanding of the pathophysiology of depression remains rudimentary.

Heterogeneity remains a major confounding factor. Until there are discriminating diagnostic markers that distinguish sub-types, treatment will remain a rather blunt instrument, exposing some to treatment that will not benefit, denying others treatment that would. Others will endure months while a succession of treatment approaches is attempted. During this time damaging morbidity and life change can occur, which then impedes recovery—until success finally results from treatment or spontaneous remission. For most people depression follows a remit-and-relapse course and with vigorous and determined treatment few will show no improvement and be chronically persistent.

Websites relevant to this chapter

Depression in adults with a chronic physical health problem: treatment and management. NICE guideline for depression with medical co-morbidities.

<www.nice.org.uk/nicemedia/pdf/CG91NICEguideline.pdf>

Depression: the treatment and management of depression in adults. CG90.

<www.nice.org.uk/nicemedia/pdf/CG90NICEguideline.pdf>

Depression. Clinical knowledge summary from NHS evidence.

<http://cls.nice.org/depression>

References

1 Ostegaard SD, Jensen SOW, Bech P. The heterogeneity of the depressive syndrome: when numbers get serious. Acta Psych Scand. 2011;**124**:495–6.

2 Koenig HG, George LK, Peterson BL, Pieper CF. Depression in medically ill hospitalized older adults: prevalence, characteristics and course of symptoms according to six diagnostic schemes. Am J Psychiat. 1997;**154**:1376–83.

3 Esquirol E. Mental maladies, a treatise on insanity. Philadelphia: Lea Blanchard; 1845.

4 Burton R. The anatomy of melancholy. London: Tegg; 1652.

5 WHO. The global burden of disease; 2004 update. Geneva: World Health Organization; 2008.

6 Moussavi S, Chatterji S, Verdes E, et al. Depression, chronic diseases, and decrements in health: results from the World Health Surveys. Lancet. 2007;**370**:851–8.

7 Van der Kooy K, Van Hout H, Marwijk H, et al. Depression and the risk for cardiovascular disease: review and meta-analysis. Int J Geriatr Psychiat. 2007;**22**:613–26.

8 National Institute for Health & Clinical Excellence. Depression in adults with a chronic physical health problem: treatment and management. CG91. National Collaborating Centre for Mental Health; 2010.

9 Ryan J, Carriere I, Ritchie K, et al. Late life depression and mortality: influence of gender and antidepressant use. Br J Psychiat. 2008;**192**:12–18.

10 Conwell Y, Dubenstein PR, Herrmann J, et al. Age differences in behaviours leading to completed suicide. Am J Geriat Psychiatry. 1998;**6**:122–6.

11 Dennis M, Wakefield P Molloy C, Andrews H, Friedman T. A study of self harm in older people: mental disorder, social factors and motives. Aging Ment Health. 2007;**11**:520–5.

12 Hawton K, Zahl D, Weartherall R. Suicide following deliberate self-harm: long-term follow-up of patients who presented to a general hospital. Br J Psychiat. 2003;**182**:537–42.

13 Hawton K, Harriss L. Deliberate self harm in people aged 60 years and over: characteristics and outcome of a 20 year cohort. Int J Geriat Psychiat. 2006;**21**:572–81.

14 Murphy E, Kapur N, Webb R, Purandare N, Hawton K, Bergen H, Waters K, Cooper J. Risk factors for repetition and suicide following self harm in older adults: multicentre cohort study. Br J Psychiat. 2012;**200**:399–404.

15 Hegeman JM, Kok RM, van der Mast, et al. Phenomenology of depression in older compared with younger adults: meta-analysis. Br J Psychiat. 2012;**200**:275–81.

16 Anderson D. Age discrimination in mental health services needs to be understood. Psychiatrist. 2011;**35**:1–4.

17 Copeland JRM, Beekman ATF, Dewey ME, et al. Depression in Europe: geographical distribution among older people. Br J Psychiat. 1999;**174**:312–21.

18 Beekman ATF, Copeland JRM, Prince MJ. Review of community prevalence of depression in later life. Br J Psychiat. 1999;**174**:307–11.

19 McCrone P, Dhanasiri S Patel A, et al. Paying the price: the cost of mental health in England to 2026. The Kings Fund; 2008.

20 Schildkraut JJ. The catecholamine hypothesis of affective disorders: a review of supporting evidence. Am J Psychiat. 1965;**122**:509–522.

21 Brown GW, Harris TO. Social origins of depression. London: Tavistock; 1978.

22 Beck AT. Cognitive therapy and the emotional disorders. New York: International Universities; 1976.

23 Prince MJ, Harwood RH, Blizard RA, Thomas A, Mann AH. Impairment, disability and handicap as risk factors for depression in old age. The Gospel Oak Project V. Psychol Med. 1997;**27**:311–21.

24 Alexopoulos GS, Meyers BS, Young RC, et al. 'Vascular depression' hypothesis. Arch Gen Psychiat. 1997;**54**:915–22.

25 Kraepelin E. Einfuhrung in die psychiatrische Klinik. [Lectures in clinical psychiatry]. 3rd English ed. Johnstone T, ed. New York: William Wood; 1901.

26 Roth M. The natural history of mental disorder in old age. J Ment Sci. 1955;**101**:281–301.

27 Sharma VK, Copeland JRM, Dewey ME, et al. Outcome of the depressed elderly living in the community in Liverpool: a 5 year follow up. Psychol Med. 1998;**28**:1329–37.

28 Licht-Strunk E, Van Marwijk HW, Hoekstra T, et al. Outcome of depression in later life in primary care: longitudinal cohort study with years follow-up. BMJ. 2009;**338**:a3079.

29 Wilson K, Mottram P, Sivananthan A, et al. Antidepressants versus placebo for the depressed elderly. Cochrane Database Syst Rev 2001;(2):CD000561.

30 **Cuijpers P**. 2007; van SA, Smit F, et al. Is psychotherapy for depression equally effective in younger and older adults? A meta regression analysis. Int Psychogeriatr. 2009:**21**;16–24.

31 **Hatcher S, Arroll B**. Newer antidepressants for the treatment of depression in adults. BMJ. 2012;**344**:1–9.

32 **Coupland C, Dhiman P, Morriss R, Arthur A, Barton G, Hippisley-Cox J.** Antidepressant use and risk of adverse outcomes in older people: population based cohort study. BMJ. 2011;**343**:d4551.

33 **National Institute for Health and Clinical Excellence**. Depression: the treatment and management of depression in adults. CG90. 2009. www.nice.org.uk/nicemedia/pdf/CG90NICEguideline.pdf

34 **Castro VM, Clements CC, Murphy SN, Gainer VS, Fava M, Weilburg JB, Erb JL, Churchill SE, Kohane IS, Losifescu DV, Smoller JW, Perlis R.** QT interval and antidepressant use: a cross sectional study of electronic records. BMJ. 2013;**346**:f288

35 **Taylor MJ, Freemantle N, Geddes JR, et al**. Early onset of selective serotonin reuptake inhibitor antidepressant action: systematic review and meta-analysis. Arch Gen Psychiat. 2006;**63**(11):1217–23.

36 **Wilkinson AM, Anderson DN, Peters S**. Age and the effects of ECT. Int J Geriatr Psychiat. 1993;**8**:401–6.

37 **Wesson ML, Wilkinson AM, Anderson DN, et al**. Does age predict the longterm outcome of depression treated with ECT? A prospective study of the longterm outcome of ECT treated depression with respect to age. Int J Geriatr Psychiat. 1997;**12**:45–52.

38 **Cooper C, Katona C, Lyketsos K, et al**. A systematic review of treatments for refractory depression in older people. Am J Psychiat. 2011;**168**:681–8.

39 **Cuijpers P, van SA, Warmerdam, L et al**. Psychotherapy versus the combination of psychotherapy and pharmacotherapy in the treatment of depression: a meta-analysis. 2009; Depress Anxiety,**26**:279–88.

40 **Old Age Depression Interest Group**. How long should the elderly take antidpressants? A double blind placebo controlled study of continuation/prophylaxis therapy with dothiepin. Br J Psychiat. 1993;**162**:175–82.

41 **Alexopoulos GS**. Depression in the elderly. Lancet. 2005;**365**:1961–70.

42 **MacDonald AJP**. Do general practitioners 'miss' depression in elderly patients? BMJ. 1986;**292**:1365–7.

43 **Watts SC, Bhutani GE, Stout IH, et al**. Mental health in older adult recipients of primary care services: is depression the key issue? Identification, treatment and the general practitioner Int J Geriatr Psychiat. 2002;**17**:427–37.

44 **Age Concern**. Improving services and support for older people with mental health problems. The second report from the UK Inquiry into Mental Health and Well-being in Later Life. 2007. http://www.ageuk.org.uk

45 **Copeland JRM, Dewey ME, Wood N, et al**. Range of mental illness among the elderly in the community: Prevalence in Liverpool using the GMS-AGECAT package. Br J Psychiat. 1997;**150**:815–23.

46 **Copeland JRM, Beekman ATF, Dewey ME, et al**. Cross-cultural comparison of depressive symptoms in Europe does not support stereotypes of ageing. Br J Psychiat. 1999;**174**:322–9.

47 Bridle C, Spanjers K, Patel S, Atherton NM, Lamb SE. Effect of exercise on depression severity in older people: systematic review and meta-analysis of randomized controlled trials. Br J Psychiat. 2012;**201**:180–5.

48 Barnett K, Mercer SW, Norbury M, et al. Epidemiology of multimorbidity and implications for health care, research and medical education: a cross sectional study. Lancet. 2012;**380**:37–43.

49 Taylor D, Meader N, Bird V, et al. Pharmacological interventions for people with depression and chronic physical health problems: systematic review and meta-analyses of safety and efficacy. Br J Psychiat. 2011;**198**:179–88.

50 Reijnders JSAM, Ehrt U, Weber WEJ, et al. A systematic review of prevalence studies of depression in Parkinson's disease. Mov Disorder. 2008;**23**:183–9.

51 National Institute for Health and Clinical Excellence. Parkinsons disease: national clinical guideline for diagnosis and management in primary and secondary care. London: Royal College of Physicians; 2006.

52 Parker G, Hadzi-Pavlovic D, Wilhelm K, et al. Defining melancholia in properties of a refined sign based measure. Br J Psychiat. 1994;**164**:316–26.

53 Johnstone ET, Deakin JF, Lawler P, et al. The Northwick Park electroconvulsive therapy trial. Lancet. 1980;**ii**:1317–20.

54 Brandon S, Cowley P, McDonald C, et al. Electroconvulsive therapy: results in depressive illness from the Leicestershire trial. BMJ. 1984;**288**:22–5.

55 Weiner RD, Coffey CE. Indications for use of electroconvulsive therapy. In: Frances AJ, Hales RE, eds. American Psychiatric Press Review, vol 7. Washington, DC: American Psychiatric Press, 1988.

56 Menza M, Dobkin RD, Marin H, et al. A controlled trial of antidepressants in patients with Parkinsons disease and depression. Neurology. 2009;**72**:886–92.

57 Tan T, Barry P, Reken S, et al. Pharmacological management of neuropathic pain in non-specialist settings: summary of NICE guidance. BMJ. 2010;**340**:c1079.

58 Barone P Scarzella L Marconi R, et al. Pramipexole versus sertraline in the treatment of depression in Parkinsons disease. J Neurol. 2006;**253**:601–7.

59 Glassman AH, O'Connor CM, Califf RM, et al. Sertraline treatment of major depression in patients with acute MI or unstable angina. JAMA-J Am Med Assoc. 2002;**288**:701–9.

60 Lesperance F, Frasure-Smith N, Koszycki D, et al. Effects of citalopram and interpersonal psychotherapy on depression in patients with coronary artery disease: the Canadian Cardiac Randomised Evaluation of Antidepressant and Psychotherapy Efficacy (CREATE) trial. JAMA-J Am Med Assoc. 2007;**297**:367–79.

61 Berkman LF, Blumenthal J, Burg M, et al. Effects of treating depression and low perceived social support on clinical events after myocardial infarction: the Enhancing Recovery in Coronary Heart Disease Patients (ENRICHD) Randomised trial. JAMA-J Am Med Assoc. 2003;**289**:3106–16.

62 Serebruany VL, Suckow RF, Cooper TB, et al. Sertraline Antidepressant Heart Attack Trial: Relationship between release of platelet/endothelial biomarkers and plasma levels of sertraline and N-desmethylsertraline in acute coronary syndrome patients receiving SSRI treatment for depression. Am J Psychiat. 2005;**162**:1165–70.

63 Price A, Rayner L, Okon-Rocha E, et al. Antidepressants for the treatment of depression in neurological disorders: a systematic review and meta-analysis of randomized controlled trials. J Neurol Neurosurg Psychiat. 2011;**82**:914–23.

64 Narushima K, Paradiso S, Moser DL, et al. Effect of antidepressant therapy on executive function after stroke. Br J Psychiat. 2007;**190**:260–5.

65 Taragano FE, Allegri R, Vicario A, et al. A double-blind randomized clinical trial assessing the efficacy and safety of augmenting standard antidepressant therapy with nimodipine in the treatment of vascular depression. Int J Geriatr Psychiat. 2001;**16**:254–60.

66 Kohler S, Thomas AJ, Lloyd A, Barber R, Almeida OP, O'Brien JT. White matter hyperintensities, cortisol levels, brain atrophy and continuing cognitive deficits in late life depression. Br J Psychiat, 2010;**196**:143–9.

67 Sirey JA, Raue PJ, Alexopoulos GS. An intervention to improve depression care in older adults with COPD. Int J Geriatr Psychiat. 2007;**22**:154–9.

68 Banerjee S, Hellier J, Dewey M, et al. Sertraline or mirtazapine for depression in dementia (HTA-SADD): a randomized, multicentre, double blind, placebo controlled trial. Lancet. 2011;**378**:403–11.

69 da Silva J, Gonsalves-Pereira M, Xavier M, et al. Affective disorders and risk of developing dementia: systematic review. Br J Psychiat. 2013;**202**:177–86.

70 Diniz BS, Butters MA, Albert SM, et al. Late-life depression and risk of vascular dementia and Alzheimer's disease: systematic review and meta-analysis of community based cohort studies. Br J Psychiat. 2013;**202**:329–35.

71 Gallo JJ, Morales KH, Bogner HR, Raue PJ, Zee J, Bruce ML, Reynolds III CF. Long term effect of depression care management on mortality in older adults: follow up of cluster randomized clinical trial in primary care. BMJ. 2013;**346**:f2570.

72 Hall WD, Mant A, Mitchell PB, Rendle VA, Hickie IB, McManus P. Association between antidepressant prescribing and suicide in Australia, 1991–2000: trend analysis. BMJ. 2003;**326**:1008.

73 Cipriani A, Hawton K, Stockton S, Geddes JR. Lithium in the prevention of suicide in mood disorders: updated systematic review and meta-analysis. BMJ. 2013;**346**:f3646.

74 Firbank MJ, Teodorczuk A, van der Fler WM, Gouw AA, Wallin A, Erkinjuntii T, Inzitari D, Wahlund L-O, Pantoni L, Pogessi A, Pracucci G, Langhorne P, O'Brien JT. Relationship between progression of brain white matter changes and late-life depression: 3 year results from the LADIS study. Br J Psychiat. 2012;**201**:40–5.

75 Dufouil C, Chalmers J, Coskun O, Besancon V, Bousser M-G, Guillon P, et al. Effects of blood pressure lowering on cerebral white matter hyperintensities in patients with stroke: the PROGRESS (Perindopril Protection Against Recurrent Stroke Study) magnetic resonance imaging substudy). Circulation. 2005;**112**:1644–50.

76 Firbank MJ, Wiseman RM, Burton EJ, Saxby BK, O'Brien JT, Ford GA. Brain atrophy and white matter hyperintensity change in older adults and relationship to blood pressure. J Neurol. 2007;**254**:713–21.

77 Mangin D, Heath I, Jamoulle M. Beyond diagnosis: rising to the multimorbidity challenge. BMJ. 2012;**344**:e3526.

Chapter 10

Substance misuse and older people: a question of values

Ilana Crome

Key points

- Substances are drugs that alter mental state and are potentially addictive.
- Substance abuse is not confined to the younger population; it is also prevalent in older people—alcohol and prescription drugs are the most commonly misused in this population.
- The possibility of substance misuse should not be dismissed because of the patient's age.
- Recommended alcohol limits are likely to be lower than for younger adults.
- Risk factors differ for older people, e.g. bereavement, retirement, loneliness, boredom.
- Substance misuse is often accompanied by other mental and physical disorders.
- Older people can improve with treatment so should be comprehensively assessed and offered evidence-based treatment regimes that are adjusted to take their special needs into account.

1 Introduction

Substances (Box 10.1) may be used appropriately (e.g. alcohol consumption within recommended 'safe' limits or medications taken as advised) or misused (taken illegally or against medical advice; e.g. smoking tobacco). Although use and misuse may have consequences for the user, regular, heavy, and risky use may result in dependence or addiction in all age groups including older people.

Box 10.1 Definition of substance and substance misuse

- In this chapter, 'substance' is used to describe licit substances (tobacco and alcohol) and illicit substances (opiates and opioids such as heroin and methadone, stimulants such as cocaine, amphetamine, and ecstasy). The term is also used to describe use of prescription drugs or medications bought over the counter and used in a manner not in accordance with medical advice.

- The term 'older' is generally used to denote over the age of 65, but if the information is based on younger age groups, this will be stated.

Substances or substance misuse contribute to the burden of disease, are highly prevalent, and reduce life expectancy.

By 2020 older people over the age of 65 years will constitute 25% of the population in the UK. National surveys, attendances at accident and emergency units, presentations to specialist addiction services, and hospital admissions for poisoning, drug, and alcohol-related mental and physical disorders indicate that there is an increasing number of older people seeking help for substance misuse (1–4). Based on these indicators, the prediction is that the number of older substance misusers will double in the next two decades.

Substance misuse is a major financial burden in the UK due to costs incurred to the health service and the criminal justice system, as well as poor productivity in the workplace. There are also wider social costs to families, friends, and wider communities, such as homelessness or divorce, that are not included in economic estimates.

Tobacco, alcohol, and illicit drugs are three of the top eight risk factors contributing to the burden of disease in Europe. The current prevalence rates of substance use in the UK reflect this concern. Approximately 13% of older men and 12% of older women still smoke cigarettes, and smoking remains the largest cause of premature death (5). Alcohol consumption above the 'safe' or 'sensible' limits for adults is found in 20% of men and 10% women over the age of 65 (3, 6). This might well underestimate the impact on older people since the recommended 'safe' limit for adult men is 3–4 units of alcohol each day and no more than 21 units each week, while that for women is 2–3 units of alcohol each day and no more than 14 units each week. One unit is equivalent to 8 g pure alcohol. However this may not be appropriate for older people (7). Conservative estimates of the costs of substance use overall to society, and specifically for older people where available, are shown in Box 10.2.

> ## Box 10.2 Alcohol-related costs
>
> - It is estimated that alcohol costs the country approximately £21 billion per year and illicit drugs cost £15 billion per year.
> - The costs are greater for older people.
> - The costs of alcohol-related inpatient admissions in England for 55–74-year-olds (£825.6 million) were more than ten times that for 16–24-year-olds (£63.8 million).
> - Eight times (317,454) as many older people were admitted compared with younger people (54,682)·
> - Alcohol-related inpatient admissions cost £1,993.57 million, compared with A&E admissions, which cost £636.3 million.
> - The cost of male inpatient admissions (£12,784 million) was almost double that of women (£715.1 million) since more men were admitted.
>
> Source: National Information Centre. Statistics on alcohol: England 2011. Health and Social Care Information Centre. <http://www.hscic.gov.uk/pubs/alcohol11>

Furthermore, alcohol-related mortality has trebled since 1984, with the greatest rate of increase in the 55–74 year age group. The highest numbers of new presentations in drug treatment units are people over 40 years, which constitutes 17 per cent of their clients. Nearly half the medications prescribed in the NHS are for over-65-year-olds. In the adult population it is estimated that substance misuse can reduce life expectancy by up to 17 years, and if combined with a serious mental illness (which is commonly the case), by a further 13 years (8, 9).

2 Diagnosis of addiction in older people

A diagnosis of dependence (commonly referred to as 'addiction') depends on having three or more of the following criteria over the previous 12 months: tolerance, withdrawal, and relief of withdrawal, inability to control use, compulsion to use, increased time spent obtaining substances, reduction of activities or obligations due to use, and continued use despite the development of physical and psychological consequences (3). It should be noted that these criteria were developed in the adult population and therefore should be applied cautiously in older people where the quantity and frequency of use may be as relevant as dependence criteria in establishing the impact of substance use on the presentation.

2.1 Competence in the comprehensive assessment as prelude to treatment

Problematic substance use can have long-term implications; it can be complex and chronic, necessitating management in partnership with the patient and family. First, however, the condition needs to be detected. There are barriers to identification by professionals that need to be overcome. The Royal Medical Colleges are working collaboratively to ensure that all medical professionals are trained in terms of their attitudes to substance misusers, knowledge about the problem, and requisite skills to competently diagnose and treat substance misusers. A non-judgemental and non-confrontational approach is key not only in treatment but also in assessment. In order to obtain a detailed history, practitioners need to be aware of subtle atypical presentations. They also need to have a high index of suspicion and to guard against ageist perceptions, stereotyping, stigmas, and myths such as 'at their age what does it matter, that is all s/he has left, treatment does not work'.

There are several screening tools available for the detection of substance problems in older people. In busy clinical practice, the most useful are the SMAST-G (Short Michigan Alcoholism Screening Test–Geriatric version), AUDIT (Alcohol Use Disorders Identification Test), and the recently developed DAPA-PC (Drug and Alcohol Problem Assessment for Primary Care). This latter is a computerized screening system that quickly identifies problems as is a self-administered, Internet-based instrument which generates a patient profile for medical reference and presents advice for the patients. Clinicians follow up if needs be. This offers a new way forward to assess patients in the future (11).

Other useful adjuncts are the 'brown bag review' where the clinician assesses the use of prescription as well as over-the-counter medication, vitamins, topical ointments, and dietary supplements which the older person might have been using. Assessment of smoking, depression, and cognition are important components to include and will give an indication of the common co-morbidities with substance misuse.

There are distinctive features of substance problems in older people. These include increased risk of medical and psychological consequences due to increased accumulation of substances as a result of decreased metabolism and increased brain sensitivity to drugs. Since older people may be on a number of prescribed medications, there is the potential for interactions and mistakes in the dispensing and consumption. This is further complicated by the use of other drugs, such as over-the-counter medications and drugs obtained via the Internet or from family and friends. Sometimes this is done unwittingly and the user is unaware of the interactions and consequences.

The practitioner needs to find out about any erratic behaviour or change in behaviour, poor response to treatment, requests for more prescription drugs, evidence of storing and sharing drugs, personal or family history of substance problems, illegal activities, as well as any personal, legal, or occupational deficits which may have resulted from past substance problems. Social function in terms of vulnerability (e.g. financial abuse), functional abilities (e.g. activities of daily living, support from the voluntary or private section), and informal social support and social pressures (e.g. debt, substance-using carers, open drug dealing) also need to be taken into account. A comprehensive assessment is the basis for optimal management and outcome. (Ellis et al 2011).

3 Risk and consequences—the geriatric giants in the room

There are several potential trajectories to explain older people's use of substances. They might have commenced use in their teenage years, since most people who are problematic substance users start before the age of 19. Alternatively, they might have started to use problematically when at an advanced age. It has been suggested that late-onset substance misuse has different aetiological factors and probably a better prognosis than earlier onset use. There is little information on what propels older people into problematic use but some social factors include bereavement (loss of spouse, family, and friends), retirement, boredom, and loneliness. Psychiatric problems, too, may push older people into substance misuse: depression, anxiety, insomnia, cognitive dysfunction, and psychosis may lead to, or result from, intoxication and withdrawal due to substance misuse. Physical illness may also be a precipitant or a consequence of substance misuse. All the geriatric giants (Chapter 1) may be causes or consequences of substance problems and iatrogenesis is one of particular relevance.

A recent study on older people with alcohol problems presenting in primary care reported that 38.5% had sleeping problems, 24.1% had gastrointestinal symptoms, 22.5% had memory problems, 16.8% felt sad, 17.8% had trips or falls, 31.7% were on hypertensive medication, 12.7% were on non-prescription medication, 11.9% were on antidepressants, and 10.1% were on sedatives (12). A long-term follow-up study on heroin users pointed to a similar use of combinations of medications and substances, as well as poor health status (13). This reflects the multiplicity of problems and treatments that may interact to create further problems if not assessed comprehensively. Self-harm in older people is a serious risk especially when combined with physical and psychological symptoms.

4 **Treatment effectiveness and critical issues**

It is unfortunate that people with addiction problems are far less likely to receive the treatment they need than are those with conditions such as hypertension, breast cancer, or asthma, where 65%, 76%, and 54%, respectively, will be treated. Patients with alcohol dependence got the lowest level of care when 30 medical conditions were reviewed. Only 10% received appropriate care (14). Critical issues in treatment for older people include the following: what the most appropriate or patients' favoured goal may be; what motivation they may have for psychological change; to what extent they find medical advice credible; and what techniques can be adapted to their particular needs when assessment, advice, and assistance are required (15–17).

Treatment interventions are commonly separated into psychosocial and pharmacological interventions. How the latter should be nested within the five As (ask, assess, advise, assist, arrange) paradigm for treatment (18) for substance problems is of considerable importance. Safety in the administration of medication for withdrawal, for maintenance of abstinence, and for relapse prevention in the older person needs to be carefully considered. In adults it is usual to diagnose dependence prior to the administration of pharmacological agents. However, as mentioned, older people may not present with the classical symptoms of the dependence syndrome, so this rule of thumb may not apply. Furthermore, in addition to accumulating substances more readily and being more sensitive to the effect of drugs, older people may be on combinations of medications for co-morbid conditions and which may interact.

Another important point is that medications which are prescribed for substance misuse have not been tested, studied, or researched in older people specifically. The British National Formulary advises 'less than half the adult dose' for diazepam or chlordiazepoxide in the treatment of anxiety for older people. Similarly, 'caution' is advised when prescribing methadone, lofexidine, or bupropion for opiate addiction and smoking cessation. There is, however, no advice for disulfiram, buprenorphine, or nicotine replacement therapy in older people. Hence, caution is advised, and treatment should ideally be initiated by a specialist in addiction and/or geriatric medicine, whenever possible. For methadone and buprenorphine, lower doses, with frequent monitoring, is mandatory. Acamprosate, disulfiram, lofexidine, and naltrexone should be used very sparingly indeed, and nicotine replacement and bupropion only if there are no contraindications. Only specialists with expertise in addiction should initiate these drugs in older people. Treatment of physical and psychological disorders should not be neglected. Unfortunately guidelines are

Table 10.1 Pharmacological treatments

Medication	Licensed	Age limits	Specific old age
Diazepam	Alcohol withdrawal	Not in children	<half adult dose for anxiety
Chlordiazepoxide	Alcohol withdrawal	Not in children	<half adult dose for anxiety
Disulfiram	Alcohol deterrent	Not in children	None
Methadone	Opiate addiction	Not in children	Caution
Buprenorphine	Opiate addiction	>16 years	None
Lofexidine	Opiate detoxification	Not in children	Caution
NRT	Nicotine withdrawal	>18 years	None
Bupropion	Smoking cessation	>18 years	Caution

generally dictated by clinical trials in which complex patients—unrepresentative samples (such as older people) with co-morbid conditions (such as substance misuse and physical and psychological disorders)—are excluded (Chapter 16). Combined treatments are rarely studied (Table 10.1).

There has been a degree of progress in the evaluation of psychosocial interventions for the older substance misuser. A recent review (17) sought to dispel myths about the futility of treatment. Sixteen studies were analyzed: eleven on alcohol misusers, three on smokers, one on heroin addiction, and one on prescription drug misuse. Most studies were undertaken in the USA. The findings were encouraging. They indicated that there was value in treating older people with substance problems, and that physicians can help this group by providing brief advice and motivational enhancement. Older substance misusers respond positively to treatment and have the capacity to change. Furthermore, older substance misusers do as well as their younger counterparts, and may even do better. Older substance misusers improve on all measures, such as reduction in substance use, physical and mental health, and social function. They may benefit from treatment in elder-specific or adult programmes, but it was postulated that if programmes were specially tailored to their needs, they may have even better outcomes. The overall implications are that older people should be given access to treatment programmes and that age is no barrier to treatment. This might translate into a reduction in health care utilization and costs. It is predicted that there are economic benefits in treatment because interventions for addiction are highly cost-effective in comparison with other health care costs. Only longer-term treatment and evaluation can answer these important questions.

5 **The future—valuing ageing addicts**

There remains a vital need to raise awareness among the public of substance misuse in older people. The enhancement of professional training and competencies for multidisciplinary teams comprising old-age psychiatrists, geriatricians, and addiction specialists, together with their teams of nurses, psychologists, social workers, and other professionals, is not an optional extra. Resources are being wasted by under-diagnosis and inappropriate treatment. A UK-based research programme could focus on trends in substance misuse, development of tailored assessment tools and techniques, relevant diagnostic criteria, and innovations in treatment management. These include refinements in what constitutes the optimal dose of pharmacological agents and what the recommendation for a 'safe' limit of alcohol should be.

Determining whether any particular programme or intervention can be recommended over any other would be a long-term objective. In the meantime, there are sufficiently robust treatments which older people should be given the opportunity to access, even though the specific evidence base for this age group is limited. However, the evidence that is available gives grounds for optimism. Availability of NHS addiction services is a further issue of major concern since there are serious shortfalls in provision.

It is up to health professionals to acknowledge that older substance misusers have numerous factors that militate against them. They may be undermined and constrained by any or a combination of the following factors: life circumstances of isolation or poverty; past or current behaviours such as crime or having been a victim of abuse; stigma of substance misuse; status of being 'older'; low self-esteem; limited functional life skills; health difficulties; mental illness; cognitive impairment. It behoves the medical profession to treat this group with integrity, dignity, compassion, and equality.

6 **Conclusion**

Older people with substance problems are likely to increase over the next decade. Since substance use and misuse in older people are associated with a numerous medical and social problems, there are some fundamental recommendations that can implemented without delay. For example, older people should not be denied a comprehensive assessment of substance use, misuse, and dependence. This is because there is a growing body of evidence that older people do as well as their younger counterparts if offered treatment. However, treatment facilities should take account of the special needs of older people so as maximize benefits of treatment. This demands not only prioritizing facilities but also ensuring that multidisciplinary teams of health and allied professionals are trained and competent to undertake effective treatment intervention. Greater focus needs to be placed on research into the causation of misuse, prevalence, and interventions for this vulnerable group. In short, this is an area of concern to all clinicians and policymakers in the care of older people. There is enough information available to insist that detection, intervention, and appropriate care models are developed to improve the lives of this group of older people.

Websites relevant to this chapter

Alcohol Concern:

<http://www.alcoholconcern.org.uk>

Public Health England:

<https://www.gov.uk/government/organisations/public-health-england>

Drugscope:

<http://www.drugscope.org.uk>

Royal College of Psychiatrists. Delivering quality care for drug and alcohol users: the ro.les and competencies of doctors.

<http://www.rcpsych.ac.uk/publications/collegereports/cr/cr173.aspx>

Key guidelines, policy documents, and reviews

Department of Health. Misuse and dependence: guidelines on clinical management (2007).

National Collaborating Centre for Chronic Conditions. Alcohol use disorders: diagnosis and clinical management of alcohol-related physical complications. NICE Clinical Practice Guideline 100. (2010)

National Collaborating Centre for Mental Health. Alcohol use disorders: diagnosis, assessment and management of harmful drinking and alcohol dependence. National Clinical Practice Guideline 115. (2011)

<http://guidance.nice.org.uk>

National Collaborating Centre for Mental Health. Drug misuse: psychosocial interventions. NICE Clinical Practice Guideline 51. (2007a)

National Collaborating Centre for Mental Health. Drug misuse: opioid detoxification. NICE Clinical Practice Guideline 52. (2007b)

Ellis et al. (11). Meta-analysis of trials of comprehensive geriatric assessment. (2011)

References

1 **European Monitoring Centre for Drugs and Drug Addiction**. Substance use among older adults: a neglected problem. Drugs in Focus (2008; issue 18). Accessed 16 Sep

2013. http://www.emcdda.europa.eu/attachements.cfm/att_50566_EN_
TDAD08001ENC_web.pdf

2 **National Treatment Agency for Substance Misuse.** Drug treatment in 2009–10.
National Treatment Agency, 2010. Accessed 15 Sep 2013. http://www.nta.nhs.uk/
uploads/nta_annualreport_0910.pdf

3 **Crome I, Rao T, Tarbuck A, Dar K, Janikiewicz S.** Our invisible addicts. 2011. Accessed
15 Sep 2013. http://www.rcpsych.ac.uk/publications/collegereports/cr/cr165.aspx

4 **Han B, Gfroerer JC, Colliver JD, Penne MA.** Substance use disorder among older
adults in the United States in 2020. Addiction. 2009;**104**(1):88–96.

5 **Seymour R, Booth L.** Statistics on smoking. Commons Library Standard Note. House of
Commons, 2010. Accessed 16 Sep 2013. http://www.parliament.uk/briefing-papers/
SN03312

6 **National Information Centre.** Statistics on alcohol: England, 2010. Health and Social
Care Information Centre, 2010. Accessed 16 Sep 2013. http://www.hscic.gov.uk/pubs/
alcohol10

7 **Crome I, Li TK, Rao R, Wu LT.** Alcohol limits in older people. Addiction.
2012;**107**(9):1541–3.

8 **Chang CK, Hayes RD, Broadbent M, Fernandes AC, Lee W, et al.** All-cause mortality
among people with serious mental illness (SMI), substance use disorders, and depressive
disorders in southeast London: a cohort study. BMC Psychiat. 2010;**10**:77.

9 **Chang CK, Hayes RD, Perera G, Broadbent MT, Fernandes AC, et al.** Life expectancy
at birth for people with serious mental illness and other major disorders from a
secondary mental health care case register in London. PLoS One. 2011;**6**(5):e19590.

10 **Naegle MA.** Screening for alcohol use and misuse in older adults: using the Short
Michigan Alcoholism Screening Test—Geriatric Version. Am J Nurs. 2008;**108**(11):
50–8.

11 **Ellis G, Whitehead MA, Robinson D, O'Neill D, Langhorne, P.** Comprehensive
geriatric assessment for older adults admitted to hospital: meta-analysis of randomised
controlled trials. BMJ. 2011;**343**:d6553.

12 **Moore AA, Blow FC, Hoffing M, Welgreen S, Davis JW, et al.** Primary care-based
intervention to reduce at-risk drinking in older adults: a randomized controlled trial.
Addiction. 2011;**106**(1):111–20.

13 **Hser YI, Hoffman V, Grella CE, Anglin MD.** A 33-year follow-up of narcotics addicts.
Arch Gen Psychiat. 2001;**58**(5):503–8.

14 **McGlynn EA, Asch SM, Adams J, Keesey J, Hicks J, et al.** The quality of health care
delivered to adults in the United States. N Engl J Med. 2003;**348**(26):2635–45.

15 **US Department of Health and Human Services.** Substance abuse among older adults.
1998. Treatment Improvement Protocol (TIP) Series 26(98-3179).

16 **Lingford-Hughes AR, Welch S, Peters L, Nutt DJ.** BAP updated guidelines: evidence-
based guidelines for the pharmacological management of substance abuse, harmful use,
addiction and comorbidity: recommendations from BAP. J Psychopharmacol.
2012;**26**(7):899–952.

17 **Moy I, Crome P, Crome I, Fisher M.** Systematic and narrative review of treatment for
older people with substance problems. Eur Geriat Med. 2011;**2**(4):212–36.

18 **Raw M, McNeill A, West R.** Smoking cessation guidelines for health professionals.
A guide to effective smoking cessation interventions for the health care system. Health
Education Authority. Thorax. 1998;**53**(Suppl 5, Pt 1):S1–19.

Chapter 11

Sleep in older people

Joe Harbison

Key points

- Sleep structure and pattern change with age, sleep typically becoming lighter and more fragmented.
- While sleep disorders may not be independently associated with age, they occur more commonly in older people due to co-morbidity.
- Common 'minor' medical conditions may seriously impair sleep quality.
- Neurological conditions such as stroke, Parkinson's, and dementia are often associated with sleep disorders which can be difficult to treat.
- Circadian rhythm disorders are common in older people; primary insomnia is rare.
- Respiratory sleep disorders are also common but their significance in many people is uncertain.
- Effective treatments are available for restless legs syndrome and related disorders.

1 Introduction

Sleep is an essential physiological process. Neural activity consistent with sleep has been found in animals as simple as the nematode, and no higher animal, to our knowledge, has evolved to the point where it no longer requires sleep. Even creatures such as migrating birds and marine mammals sleep despite the challenges of doing so while flying or swimming.

However, the actual purpose of sleep is still controversial in some respects. In young mammals' sleep, particularly, rapid eye movement (REM) sleep plays an ontogenetic role in brain and cognitive development. Sleep deprivation in early life can result in behavioural disturbances and even reduction in brain mass in animal models (1–3). Sleep probably has an anabolic and restorative function. Animals suffering prolonged sleep deprivation show an impairment of immune function and those forcibly kept awake have shown immune failure with time. Another restorative function of sleep is in the healing of tissue injury, but it is unclear whether healing occurs faster at night for any reason other than relative immobilization of injured tissue.

Sleep has an important role in processing and recording of memory in humans, although the specifics of the relationship remain controversial. Sleep seems to facilitate the sorting and either retention or 'unlearning' of memories that have been accumulated in the recent past. REM sleep appears to have a role in procedural and spatial memory, and, some have suggested, a role in the unconscious 'rehearsal' of motor activities. Non-REM, slow-wave sleep appears to have a role in the retention of declarative memory; i.e. memory for facts and figures (semantic memory) and memory for life events (episodic memory). Normal sleep structure changes and evolves throughout the life cycle and in older humans is influenced by numerous physiological, environmental, and pathological factors.

2 Normal sleep in older people

A number of changes in sleep structure and pattern are commonly seen in older people. Whether these changes are truly physiological or are actually pathological but occurring in a very high proportion of the older population is debated. Across an adult lifespan, in healthy individuals, total sleep time decreases by anything up to 90–120 minutes (4) per night. Sleep efficiency—the time in any sleep period spent asleep rather than awake—diminishes, and sleep may become more polyphasic. Sleep becomes more easily interrupted by external stimuli, and periods of wakefulness during sleep become more prolonged. Sleep latency—the time taken to fall asleep—generally remains unchanged, but this is strongly influenced by sleep deprivation in all age groups. Proportion of light stage 1 and 2 sleep increases with age and is matched by a corresponding decrease in deep stage 3 and 4 sleep. Duration of REM sleep declines with declining sleep time, but its proportion of the total is usually maintained. REM sleep latency—the delay from sleep onset to REM sleep—is unchanged. What is perhaps most interesting is that these changes in sleep structure appear to develop in people's youth and middle age, whereas beyond 60 years there is little change in sleep structure except for a slight (3% per decade) further reduction in sleep efficiency.

It is worth emphasizing that these alterations in sleep pattern are what occurs in healthy subjects and that sleep is profoundly affected by other disease states. Ageing per se is not associated with an increased risk of sleep disorders (5) but is associated with development of frailty and both medical and psychological conditions that impact on sleep. Reported prevalence of sleep disorders in older people varies greatly depending on definitions used and method of study. In the US, sleep disorders are reported by more than 50% of community-dwelling elders and more than two thirds of those in institutional care (6, 7). Sleep disorders and disturbance also frequently contribute to decisions to place older people in institutional care, with between 70 and 80% of carers reporting their own sleep disturbance as influencing their decision (7). Sleep disorders in older people have been reported associated with increased risk of falls, decreased quality of life, and increased mortality (8–10). There may also be an association between sleep disorders, particularly respiratory sleep disorders, and the development of adult onset diabetes. The association was first noted for sleep-disordered breathing (11), but it is now suspected that the association may exist with non-respiratory sleep disorders (12).

3 Common medical and psychiatric disorders and sleep

Sleep disorders in older people commonly occur secondary to other medical conditions. Symptoms, which may be perceived as being 'minor' by medical practitioners or relatives, may be enough to significantly disrupt the sleep of an older person to the extent where it affects quality of life and daytime functioning. Examples of such symptoms include gastro-oesophageal reflux, arthritic or neuropathic pain, chronic cough, and nocturia. Poorly controlled diabetes may result in a sufficient nocturnal polyuria to adversely affect sleep quality.

Common neurological conditions can also have direct effects on sleep structure. In the days immediately following stroke, subjects can completely lose the ability to generate REM sleep (13, 14). In the longer term, more than 50% suffer from insomnia and more than one quarter may suffer daytime sleepiness (15, 16). Parasomnias such as restless legs syndrome are also commoner following stroke (17).

Nearly two thirds of people with Parkinson's disease report sleep problems, twice the rate in control populations (18), and sleep disorders are found in 74–89% of subjects on formal investigation (19). This may be influenced directly by the effect on dopaminergic pathways, which may precipitate sudden sleep attacks, but also indirectly by the immobility associated with the disease and the medications used to treat it. Insomnia, circadian rhythm disorders, parasomnias (as described later in the chapter), and daytime sleepiness are all much more common in individuals with Parkinson's disease.

Most dementing processes are associated with changes in sleep pattern and structure. Between 40% and 70% of people with dementia have a concomitant sleep disorder on evaluation. Perhaps the most recognized of these among geriatricians is the increasing agitation and confusion suffered by about 10–20% of people with dementia in the late evening, described as 'sundowning'. This is worsened by the progression of polyphasic sleep and frequent daytime naps in this population as circadian rhythm deteriorates. The evidence for treating sleep disorders in the group is very limited and thus there is widespread use of agents such as antipsychotics and benzodiazepines to help manage the problems. In reality this use is frequently ineffective in improving sleep quality and is actually employed as a means of pharmaceutical restraint. Such use increases risk of falls and fracture and increases mortality (20, 21). Prior to consideration of hypnotic treatment, other interventions can be considered, including behaviour modification; prevention of excessive daytime sleeping; provision of stimulants to wakefulness at appropriate times, such as exposure to bright light in the morning; being taken outside for walks; and establishment and maintenance of a definite daytime routine of rising, dressing, mealtimes at table, etc. While commonly advocated, few of these non-pharmacological therapies have been subjected to robust clinical trials (22). There may be some evidence for the use of melatonin in people with sundowning and delerium (23), although previous studies have failed to show improvement of sleep in institutionalized Alzheimer's patients with this medication (24). Studies have been small and a larger definitive trial is needed.

Anxiety and depressive disorders are common in older people (10–20% prevalence of each) and it is important to remember that new or recent onset sleep disorder in an older person may be an indicator of the development of neuropsychiatric disease (25–27). The evidence for the effect on sleep quality of treatment of anxiety disorder in older people using anxiolytics is limited. Antidepressants can have complex effects on sleep structure and quality which vary depending on mechanism of action. The newer antidepressant agomelatine, is a melatonin receptor agonist and selective serotonin receptor antagonist and may be superior to selective serotonin reuptake inhibitors in improving sleep quality in subjects with depression (28). Unfortunately, the effects of agomelatine have not been assessed in subjects with dementia and its use is therefore currently restricted to non-demented subjects.

Even where diseases themselves do not cause a sleep disorder, their treatment may. A large proportion of medications have 'sleep disorders' listed as potential adverse effects. Commonly used agents to be aware of include corticosteroids, thyroid drugs, angiotensin-converting enzyme inhibitors and statins, all of which have been reported to cause insomnia. Patients prescribed diuretics for hypertension or oedema often complain of insomnia precipitated by nocturia. Even antihistamines, generally accepted as sedating and occasionally used as hypnotics, can cause a paradoxical arousal in a minority of patients. Beta blockers cause disturbing dreams as do leukotriene receptor antagonists, such as montelukast prescribed for asthma. Other commonly used drugs such as tobacco, caffeine, and alcohol may significantly impair sleep quality but are often forgotten when looking for the cause of sleep disturbance.

4 Insomnia and circadian rhythm disorders

Circadian rhythms that dictate the levels of wakefulness and sleepiness in mammals are controlled by the tiny suprachiasmatic nucleus (SCN). With ageing, and particularly in people with neurodegenerative conditions such as Alzheimer's disease, outputs from the SCN lose synchronization and periodicity and become less effective in modulating arousal level. Thus circadian rhythm disorders are common in older subjects. The commonest disorders seen in older adults are irregular sleep-wake rhythms, particularly in patients with neurodegenerative disease and in those in long-term care with inadequate 'zeitgebers'—triggers for time and expected sleep-wake status such as clocks, regular mealtimes, and exposure to bright light. Advanced sleep phase disorder (ASPD), where an individual begins to fell sleepy early in the evening but awakens early in the morning, is also more common among older people. Delayed sleep phase disorder is commoner among teenagers and adolescents. Extrinsic circadian rhythm disorders such as jet lag and shift work disorder tend to affect older people more severely. Circadian rhythm disorders are frequently misdiagnosed as insomnia and treated with sedatives, which can actually worsen the problem by further attenuating the effect of the SCN. Recommended treatments include exposing people to daylight or bright light at appropriate times of the day, improving sleep hygiene by reintroducing a daily and bedtime routine and, in the case of ASPD, gradually delaying bedtime by one hour weekly until a normal sleep phase is regained (29, 30).

The prevalence of insomnia varies hugely between studies and depending on the method used to diagnose it. Primary insomnia developing in old age is very rare. Insomnia is therefore usually due to an underlying medical, environmental, or psychological problem. When investigating insomnia it is important to take a detailed history and determine if the person is getting too little sleep or has unrealistic expectations of how much sleep they should be getting. An absence of significant daytime sleepiness is an indicator that they may be getting enough normal sleep. An effort should then be made to determine how much sleep the person is getting in a day and whether in fact they have a circadian rhythm disorder. A collateral history is valuable as many people underestimate how much sleep they get, particularly if they have an underlying cognitive disorder. Management should be to identify, as far as possible, the underlying cause of the problem and to remove it. Emphasis should be given to sleep hygiene as previously described, avoidance of caffeine and other stimulants in the afternoon and evening, and avoidance of using their bed to watch television, read, eat, etc. Sleeping tablets such as GABAA receptor agonists (Z drugs) or benzodiazepines should not be used except where the insomnia is severely distressing or disabling and for periods not exceeding two weeks. It is worth emphasizing that sleeping tablets have roughly twice the chance of producing an unwanted side effect (e.g. falls or cognitive impairment) as they have of delivering an improved night sleep (20).

5 Sleep-disordered breathing

Sleep-disordered breathing, in particular obstructive sleep apnoea (OSA), is very common in older people. More than 55% of subjects over 70 years in the large Sleep Heart Health Study had an apnoea-hypopnoea index >5 (31), a finding that has been supported by other studies (32). The challenge in these results is that we are still unsure as to the significance of OSA in this population. Presence of obstructive apnoea in sleep studies is not the same as the clinical phenomenon of obstructive sleep apnoea syndrome (OSAS) in which loud snoring, apnoeas, and consequent arousals from sleep result in profound daytime sleepiness. OSAS is also associated with hypertension and increased risk of cardiovascular disease. Older people are less likely to show daytime sleepiness associated with frequent apnoeas and are also less likely to have the associated loud snoring. We also lack evidence for the independent association between severity of OSA and adverse cardiovascular events in this population. The typical lack of sleepiness in older people is important in consideration of treatment, as severity of daytime sleepiness is the strongest predictor of compliance with standard nasal continuous positive airway pressure (nCPAP) treatment. Frequency of apnoeas during sleep correlates with extent of white matter disease (33) and severity of apnoeas may simply be a marker for this or for frailty (34). Certainly the nature and direction of the association between age and sleep-disordered breathing remains in question. However, if a patient presents with symptoms of OSAS they should be considered for evaluation for active therapy including nCPAP, if tolerated.

6 Parasomnias

The parasomnias are a broad group of sleep disorders characterized by abnormal or unusual behaviours, movements, or perceptions that can be associated with sleep. They can occur on falling asleep, on awakening, and during or between sleep stages. Perhaps the most familiar parasomnia is the hypnic jerk or 'sleep start' that frequently affects people as a sudden shock or arousal on falling asleep and is thought to be due to a failure to enter stage 2 from stage 1 sleep.

The commonest parasomnias that present to geriatricians are nocturnal leg cramps and restless legs syndrome, previously known as Ekbom's syndrome. Nocturnal leg cramps affect one in three people over 60 years and half of 80-year-olds (35). In most cases the cause is unclear but they can be associated with peripheral vascular disease, renal failure, cirrhosis, electrolyte disturbances, or hypothyroidism, and evaluation of these is advisable if the symptoms appear or deteriorate suddenly. Commonly used medications, which may worsen cramps, include statins, diuretics, nifedipine, and nicotinic acid. Suggested treatment involves identifying and resolving underlying causes and then advising simple measures such as calf stretching exercises before bedtime. Avoiding circumstances where the calf muscles are in forced flexion during the night is advisable and avoiding tucking in blankets and sheets at the bottom may help (36). Although evidence for such actions is lacking (37), they may help, and are unlikely to cause the condition to deteriorate or have significant side effects. Quinine helps reduce frequency of attacks in those severely affected, but it has a number of potentially unpleasant side effects (38). Particular advice needs to be given to prevent children taking quinine tablets, as a small number may lead to permanent blindness in a small child. Issues of toxicity have led to its use being cautioned against in some guidelines (36).

Restless legs syndrome (RLS) is a disorder characterized by an irresistible urge to move one's body or limbs to relieve an unpleasant sensation. This feeling is described variously as 'a crawling sensation', 'worms under the skin', or 'electric shocks'. It predominantly affects the legs and gets worse as the individual becomes drowsy. The cause is not fully understood (39), but it occurs commonly in people with Parkinson's disease, and therefore a disorder in a dopaminergic pathway is suspected. Among other disorders it is associated with iron deficiency and uraemia and these need to be ruled out in cases where the condition appears or deteriorates suddenly. Drugs such as caffeine and many antidepressants can make the symptoms worse. About 60% of cases are familial with an autosomal dominant inheritance with variable penetrance. Until recently treatment was with co-careldopa, but this frequently produced a rebound effect the following morning. Treatment has been revolutionized by the introduction of the non-ergot dopamine agonists ropinirole and pramipexole administered in low dose titrating up with effect (40). As an alternative, calcium channel alpha-2-delta ligands such as gabapentin and pregabalin are also effective in treating RLS (41).

Periodic limb movement (PLM) disorder seems to be related to RLS and may occur with it in up to 80% of cases. In PLM, people suffer sudden abrupt movements of their limbs, most typically a 'backward kick' of the legs, that can occur in intervals of 5 to 90 seconds. The movements are usually fairly minor but can be severe enough to disrupt sleep, or rarely to injure a bed partner. Treatment is essentially the same as for RLS (42).

Confusion arousals are conditions most associated with young children who are disoriented when arousing from deep sleep. They can occur in older people, especially those with an underlying cognitive impairment or taking psychotropic medications, including sleeping tablets, especially in combination with alcohol. In these episodes the individual wakes up from sleep and may seem very confused, agitated, or even aggressive or paranoid (43). This can occur when they have been asleep in informal situations; e.g. falling asleep at the television or in an airliner.

Other less common parasomnias include hypnogogic hallucinations occurring at onset of sleep and REM sleep behaviour disorder (RBD), where an individual 'acts out' their dreams. This disorder is thought to be consequent to dysfunction of the brainstem atonic pathway during REM sleep. It is frequently associated with developing neurodegenerative disease, especially Parkinson's disease (44), dementia with Lewy bodies, and multiple system atrophy. RBD is typically managed with clonazepam, which is effective in approximately 90% of cases. Melatonin may also be effective (45). Pramipexole is effective where RBD occurs in association with Parkinson's disease (46).

7 Future directions

While there is a slow increasing awareness of sleep disorders among physicians, sleep medicine is still challenged by a lack of awareness of the prevalence of sleep disorders; their association with other diseases as a symptom, cause, and complication; their effect on patients' health and quality of life; and their management and treatment. Perhaps the most important step forward needed in sleep medicine is an improvement in education and training of colleagues in the recognition, investigation, and treatment of such disorders.

We still have much to learn about the neurobiology of sleep. The fact that we have very limited understanding of the causes of such common phenomena as restless legs syndrome and sundowning reflects how much basic research is needed into sleep disorders in older people. While advances have been made in the treatment of some parasomnias such as restless legs, we still too frequently fall back on older, potentially hazardous pharmacological therapies such as benzodiazepines and quinine to manage conditions, the etiologies of which we do not understand adequately. Developing a better understanding will hopefully lead us to develop more effective and less toxic means of treating these disorders.

Respiratory sleep disorders are extremely common in older people, but we still do not fully understand their clinical relevance and if, when, and how they should be investigated and treated. We need to understand, for instance, whether sleep-disordered breathing is a cause or an effect of pathological processes in older people—or even both.

8 Conclusion

Sleep disorders are among the commonest disorders found in older people worldwide. In the last 20 years we have developed an increasing understanding of sleep in older people; however, there is still a huge amount we do not fully understand. Sleep disorders are associated with considerable morbidity, mortality, and impairment of quality of life in their own right, and are an important marker of underlying systemic disease in older people. Sleep disorders are highly prevalent in older people and our increased understanding of their relevance may earn them a place among the 'geriatric giants' of the twenty-first century.

Websites relevant to this chapter

In the absence of a robust evidence base, the Internet is awash with sites and advic.e on sleep disorders in older people. Much of the advice, unfortunately, is incorrect, misleading, or contradictory. Nevertheless, websites from the US National Sleep Foundation and the National Institute of Aging contain easily accessible advice and information on sleep and sleep disorders in older people aimed at patients and carers:

<http://www.sleepfoundation.org/article/sleep-topics/aging-and-sleep>
<http://www.nia.nih.gov/health/publication/good-nights-sleep>

The American Academy of Sleep Medicine has produced guidelines for a number of common sleep disorders that are relevant to an older population:

<http://www.aasmnet.org/practiceguidelines.aspx>

Resources and information on sleep medicine in Europe is less developed than in the US, but there is some useful information on the European Sleep Research Society and British Sleep Society's websites:

<http://www.esrs.eu/>
<http://www.sleepsociety.org.uk/>

Key guidelines, policy documents, and reviews

Apart from those produced by the American Academy of Sleep Medicine, there are limited good quality, evidence-based guidelines available, and certainly no single good resource for such. The UK National Institute of Health and Care Excellence has a number of guidelines relevant to sleep in older people. These include:

Sleep apnoea—continuous positive airway pressure (CPAP) (TA139)

Insomnia—newer hypnotic drugs (TA77)

Parkinson's disease (CG35)

Depression in adults (update) (CG90)

Depression with a chronic physical health problem (CG91)

Delirium (CG103)

Anxiety (CG113)

All are available through <www.nice.org.uk>.

References

1 Gregory AM, Sadeh A. Sleep, emotional and behavioral difficulties in children and adolescents. Sleep Med Rev. 2012;**16**:129–36.

2 Touchette E, Petit D, Tremblay RE, Montplaisir JY. Risk factors and consequences of early childhood dyssomnias: New perspectives. Sleep Med Rev. 2009;**13**:355–61.

3 Novati A, Hulshof HJ, Koolhaas JM, Lucassen PJ, Meerlo P. Chronic sleep restriction causes a decrease in hippocampal volume in adolescent rats, which is not explained by changes in glucocorticoid levels or neurogenesis. Neuroscience. 2011;**190**:145–55.

4 Ohayon MM, Carskadon MA Guilleminault C, Vitiello MV. Meta-analysis of quantitative sleep parameters from childhood to old age in healthy individuals: developing normative sleep values across the human lifespan. Sleep. 2004;**27**:1255–73.

5 Neikrug AB, Ancoli-Israel S. Sleep disorders in the older adult—a mini review. Gerontology. 2010;**56**:181–9.

6 Becker PM, Jamieson AO. Common sleep disorders in the elderly: diagnosis and treatment. Geriatrics. 1992;**47**: 41–52.

7 Pollack CP, Perlick D. Sleep problems and institutionalization of the Elderly. J Geriatr Psychiat Neurol. 1991;**4**: 204–10.

8 Stone KL, Ancoli-Israel S, Blackwell T, Ensrud KE, Cauley JA, Redline SS, Hillier TA, Schneider J, Claman D, Cummings SR. Poor sleep is associated with increased risk of falls in older women. Arch Intern Med. 2008;**168**:1768–75.

9 Schubert CR, Cruikshanks KJ, Dalton DS, Klein BE, Klein R, Nondahl DM. Prevalence of sleep problems and quality of life in an older population. Sleep. 2002;**25**:889–93.

10 Dew MA, Hoch CC, Buysse DJ, Monk TH, Begley AE, Houck P, Hall M, Kupfer D, Reynolds CF III. Healthy older adults' sleep predicts all-cause mortality at 4 to 19 years of follow-up. Psychosom Med. 2003;**65**: 63–73.

11 Shaw JE, Punjabi NM, Wilding JP, Alberti KG, Zimmet PZ. Sleep-disordered breathing and type 2 diabetes: a report from the International Diabetes Federation Taskforce on Epidemiology and Prevention. Diabetes Res Clin Pract. 2008;**81**:2–12.

12 Cappuccio FP, D'Elia L, Strazzullo P, Miller MA. Quantity and quality of sleep and incidence of type 2 diabetes: a systematic review and meta-analysis. Diabetes Care. 2010;**33**:414–20.

13 Hachinski VC, Mamelak M, Norris JW. Clinical recovery and sleep architecture degradation. Can J Neurol Sci. 1990;**17**:332–5.

14 Giubilei F, Iannilli M, Vitale A, Pierallini A, Sacchetti ML, Antonini G, Fieschi C. Sleep patterns in acute ischemic stroke. Acta Neurol Scand. 1992;**86**:567–71.

15 Leppavuori A, Pohjasvaara T, Vataja R, Kaste M, Erkinjuntti T. Insomnia in ischemic stroke patients. Cerebrovasc Dis. 2002;**14**: 90–7.

16 Hermann DM, Bassetti CL. Sleep-related breathing and sleep-wake disturbances in ischemic stroke. Neurology. 2009;**73**:1313–22.

17 Lee SJ, Kim JS, Song IU, An JY, Kim YI, Lee KS. Poststroke restless legs syndrome and lesion location: anatomical considerations. Mov Disord. 2009;**24**:77–84.

18 Tandberg E, Larsen JP, Karlsen K. A community-based study of sleep disorders in patients with Parkinson's disease. Mov Disord. 1998;**13**:895–9.

19 Garcia-Borreguero D, Larrosa O, Bravo M. Parkinson's disease and sleep. Sleep Med Rev. 2003;**7**:115–29.

20 Glass J, Lanctot KL, Hermann N, Sproule BA, Busto UE. Sedative hypnotics in older people with insomnia: meta-analysis of risks and benefits. BMJ. 2005;**331**:1169.

21 Schneider LS, Dagerman KS, Insel P. Risk of death with atypical antipsychotic drug treatment for dementia: meta-analysis of randomized placebo-controlled trials. JAMA-J Am Med Assoc. 2005;**294**:1934–43.

22 Khachiyants N, Trinkle D, Son SJ, Kim KY. Sundown syndrome in persons with dementia: an update. Psychiat Investig. 2011;**8**:275–87.

23 Al-Aama T, Brymer C, Gutmanis I, Woolmore-Goodwin SM, Esbaugh J, Dasgupta M. Melatonin decreases delirium in elderly patients: A randomized, placebo-controlled trial. Int J Geriatr Psychiat. 2011;**26**:687–94.

24 Gehrman PR, Connor DJ, Martin JL, Shochat T, Corey-Bloom J, Ancoli-Israel S. Melatonin fails to improve sleep or agitation in double-blind randomized placebo-controlled trial of institutionalized patients with Alzheimer disease. Am J Geriat Psychiat. 2009;**17**:166–9.

25 Spira AP, Stone K, Beaudreau SA, Ancoli-Israel S, Yaffe K. Anxiety symptoms and objectively measured sleep quality in older women. Am J Geriat Psychiat. 2009;**17**:136–43.

26 Maglione JE, Ancoli-Israel S, Peters KW, Paudel ML, Yaffe K, Ensrud KE, Stone KL. Depressive symptoms and subjective and objective sleep in community-dwelling older women. J Am Geriatr Soc. 2012;**60**:635–43.

27 Spiegelhalder K, Regen W, Nanovska S, Baglioni C, Riemann D. Comorbid sleep disorders in neuropsychiatric disorders across the life cycle. Curr Psychiat Rep. 2013;**15**: 364.

28 Corruble E, de Bodinat C, Belaïdi C, Goodwin GM. Efficacy of agomelatine and escitalopram on depression, subjective sleep and emotional experiences in patients with major depressive disorder: a 24-wk randomized, controlled, double-blind trial. Int J Neuropsychopharmacol. 2013;**3**:1–16.

29 Morgenthaler TI, Lee-Chiong T, Alessi C, Friedman L, Aurora RN, Boehlecke B, Brown T, Chesson AL Jr, Kapur V, Maganti R, Owens J, Pancer J, Swick TJ, Zak R. Practice parameters for the clinical evaluation and treatment of circadian rhythm sleep disorders. Sleep. 2007;**30**:1445–59.

30 Sack RL, Auckley D, Auger RR, Carskadon MA, Wright KP Jr, Vitiello MV, Zhdanova IV. Circadian rhythm sleep disorders: part II, advanced sleep phase disorder, delayed sleep phase disorder, free-running disorder, and irregular sleep-wake rhythm. Sleep. 2007;**30**:1484–501.

31 Young T, Shahar E, Nieto FJ, Redline S, Newman AB, Gottlieb DJ, Walsleben JA, Finn L, Enright P, Samet JM; Sleep Heart Health Study Research Group. Predictors of sleep-disordered breathing in community dwelling adults: the sleep heart study. Arch Int Med. 2002;**162**:893–900.

32 Ancoli-Israel S, Gehrman P, Kripke DF, Stepnowsky C, Mason W, Cohen-Zion M, Marler M. Long-term follow up of sleep disordered breathing in older adults. Sleep Med. 2001;**2**:511–6.

33 Harbison J, Gibson GJ, Birchall D, Zammit-Maempel I, Ford GA. White matter disease and sleep-disordered breathing following stroke. Neurology. 2003;**61**:959–63.

34 Endeshaw YW, Unruh ML, Kutner M, Newman AB, Bliwise DL. Sleep-disordered breathing and frailty in the Cardiovascular Health Study Cohort. Am J Epidemiol. 2009;**170**:193–202.

35 Butler JV, Mulkerrin EC, O'Keeffe ST. Nocturnal leg cramps in older people. Postgrad Med J. 2002;**78**:596–8.

36 Allen RE, Kirby KA. Nocturnal leg cramps. Am Fam Physician. 2012;**86**:350–5.

37 Blyton F, Chuter V, Walter KE, Burns J. Non-drug therapies for lower limb muscle cramps. Cochrane Database Syst Rev. 2012 Jan 18;**1**:CD008496.

38 Townend BS, Sturm JW, Whyte S. Quinine associated blindness. Aust Fam Physician. 2004;**33**:627–8.

39 Trenkwalder C, Paulus W. Restless legs syndrome: pathophysiology, clinical presentation and management. Nat Rev Neurol. 2010;**6**:337–46.

40 Garcia-Borreguero D, Kohnen R, Silber MH, Winkelman JW, Earley CJ, Högl B, Manconi M, Montplaisir J, Inoue Y, Allen RP. The long-term treatment of restless legs syndrome/Willis-Ekbom disease: evidence-based guidelines and clinical consensus best practice guidance: a report from the International Restless Legs Syndrome Study Group. Sleep Med. 2013;**14**:675–84.

41 Wilt TJ, MacDonald R, Ouellette J, Khawaja IS, Rutks I, Butler M, Fink HA. Pharmacologic therapy for primary restless legs syndrome: a systematic review and meta-analysis. JAMA Intern Med. 2013;**173**:496–505.

42 Aurora RN, Kristo DA, Bista SR, Rowley JA, Zak RS, Casey KR, Lamm CI, Tracy SL, Rosenberg RS. The treatment of restless legs syndrome and periodic limb movement disorder in adults-an update for 2012: practice parameters with an evidence-based systematic review and meta-analyses. Sleep. 2012;**35**:1039–62.

43 Stores G. Dramatic parasomnias. J R Soc Med. 2001 April;**94**(4):173–6.

44 Boeve BF. Idiopathic REM sleep behaviour disorder in the development of Parkinson's disease. Lancet Neurol. 2013;**12**:469–82.

45 McCarter SJ, Boswell CL, St Louis EK, Dueffert LG, Slocumb N, Boeve BF, Silber MH, Olson EJ, Tippmann-Peikert M. Treatment outcomes in REM sleep behavior disorder. Sleep Med. 2013;**14**:237–42.

46 Aurora RN, Zak RS, Maganti RK, Auerbach SH, Casey KR, Chowdhuri S, Karippot A, Ramar K, Kristo DA, Morgenthaler TI. Standards of Practice Committee. Best practice guide for the treatment of REM sleep behavior disorder (RBD). J Clin Sleep Med. 2010;**6**:85–95.

Chapter 12

Assessment and management of pain in older adults

Pat Schofield

Key points

- Chronic persistent pain affects at least 50% of community-dwelling older adults.

- Physiological changes that occur as a result of the ageing process need to be considered when dealing with pain in the older adult.

- Assessment of pain can be complicated when the older adult is unable to articulate their pain; for example, in the presence of cognitive impairment.

- Much of the research into pain management has been carried out among the younger population and simply translated across.

1 Introduction

Evidence suggests that pain is a common problem for older people, with chronic persistent pain affecting at least 50% of community-dwelling older adults. Pain foci most often cited in prevalence studies are knees, hips, and back. It is believed that the incidence of pain in the oldest and most vulnerable people, such as those living in care homes, increases to 80%.

2 Chronic and acute pain

Cancer is the second leading cause of death for adults over the age of 65 years (1) and it has been suggested that approximately 26% of cancer patients over the age of 65 years suffering daily pain did not receive any analgesic agent (2); thus both chronic and cancer pain control is an issue for the older population. It is important to differentiate between these two major classifications as management is very different. Often there is the assumption that chronic pain is part of getting older and something that the individuals must learn to live with. Nevertheless, we are seeing increasing publications on chronic pain management for older adults and there is a growing awareness that self-management of chronic pain is a viable strategy for this population (3).

Chronic pain is something that exists beyond the expected healing time and is something that often has no identifiable physical cause (4). Acute pain, on the other hand, is a sign of injury or disease, is treatable or even curable and as such, it would be expected that older adults would fare better with the management of acute pain. Yet Desbiens et al. (5) demonstrated that 46% of older people admitted to hospital report pain and 19% of these individuals have moderate or extremely severe pain; 13% were dissatisfied with their pain management.

3 Pain management

Why is pain so difficult to manage in our older population?

It has been suggested that admission to hospital for patients over the age of 65 years is three times higher than their younger counterparts and that professionals tend to underestimate pain needs, underprescribe, and undermedicate (6). We may assume that with high numbers of older adults seen in hospital, staff would be more experienced in dealing with their specific problems; in particular, more skilled in the techniques associated with assessment and management of pain. Unfortunately this is not the case. Negative attitudes to pain management in the older adult among health professionals pervade, with fears and misconceptions regarding interaction between pre-existing co-morbidities and the prescription of analgesic drugs. Such concerns are not totally unfounded as older adults are also likely to have diminished functional status and physiological reserve, as well age-related pharmacodynamic and pharmacokinetic changes (7). Furthermore, cognitive impairment can prevent pain assessment being carried out.

Ageist attitudes towards the older adult may exist: we assume they get used to pain or it is a natural part of ageing. We also know that health care professionals become desensitized to pain as they become more experienced.

4 Physiological function and ageing

Some changes that occur within the anatomy and physiology are considered a normal part of the ageing process; these have been discussed in other chapters. However in relation to pain, there are a number of important considerations. There is an age-related reduction in β endorphin content and GABA synthesis in the lateral thalamus, and a lower concentration of GABA and serotonin receptors. There is an age-related capacity or speed of processing of nociceptive stimuli and c and Aδ fibre function decreases with age (8). The potential for cognitive impairment increases with age and this is aggravated by pain and pain medications. Of particular note is the new belief that respiratory depression associated with opioids is more likely to be a result of the higher plasma concentration of opioids rather than a sensitivity to the respiratory depressant effects, as previously thought (9).

Ageing is also associated with a reduction in renal plasma flow of about 10% per decade (10) and a decrease in liver mass annually of about 1% (11). As discussed by Jackson in Chapter 5, hepatic and renal function changes can lead to altered clearances of medications that may lead to increased sensitivity to drugs, including pain medications.

4.1 **Pain threshold**

There has been much debate within the literature as to whether or not pain perception threshold increases with age. Gibson and Farrell (12) suggest that the threshold for pain is increased in older people when the stimuli are shorter, are distributed over a lower spatial extent, or are presented at peripheral cutaneous or visceral sites. Similarly, Helme et al. (13) suggested that older adults have an increased threshold for thermal and electrically induced pain.

However, more recent studies by Farrell (14) propose that pain is present in the same format regardless of age. Thus the experience of pain is exactly the same regardless of age; it is the perception and consequential behaviours that may vary. So pain in the older adult is influenced by both intrinsic factors, such as physiological changes, and extrinsic factors, such as barriers, attitudes, and beliefs of health care professionals.

5 **Dementia and pain**

As mentioned earlier, adults over the age of 80 are more likely to experience pain and also are more likely to have cognitive impairment, which can prohibit effective pain assessment and management. This has been demonstrated in a study by Conway and Schofield (15) who showed that in 368 care homes in one area, of more than 10,000 residents, more than 6,000 had dementia. Pain often presents as 'challenging behaviour' in this group, and can be reduced significantly by using simple analgesics such as paracetamol (16). Where individuals are unable to verbalize pain, behavioural tools can be used as a surrogate measure.

As our population ages, there will be increased numbers of adults with dementias. This can be problematic for the patient who may no longer be able to articulate their pain in a language that we can understand. So typical pain assessment measures may not be applicable and we may have to resort to behavioural scales.

6 **The assessment of pain**

In September 1990 the Royal College of Surgeons and the College of Anaesthetists published the report of their working party, 'Pain after Surgery' (17). This report can be accessed from any library or anaesthetic department and makes recommendations regarding the management of post-operative pain in the UK. These recommendations have been implemented widely and have significantly changed all aspects of pain management. One of the key recommendations was that assessment of pain should be recorded along with other routine observations such as blood pressure and pulse. The Joint Commission on Accreditation of Healthcare Organizations (18) also suggests that pain should be recognized as the fifth vital sign. The multidimensional character of pain is emphasized by the National Guidelines for Assessment of Pain for Older People (19), which describe pain at several levels:

- the sensory dimension: the intensity, location, and character of the pain sensation
- the affective dimension: the emotional component of pain and how pain is perceived
- its impact: the disabling effects of pain on the person's ability to function and participate in society.

A review of the literature related to pain assessment highlighted 42 articles written since 1995 that use various pain assessment tools with the older adult (20). From this work it can be seen that there has been very little research related to older adults and there is a need for more work to be carried out in order to investigate the most appropriate tools. Generally it has been found that this age group prefers the verbal descriptors (none, mild, moderate, severe) or the numerical rating scale, which can be accessed from the British Pain Society website (<http://www.britishpainsociety.org/>) (21). Interestingly, the literature suggests that the faces scale is not popular with this age group as the facial expressions are associated with mood. Clearly more research is needed in this area.

In summary, the numerical rating scale and the verbal descriptor scale are the most appropriate to measure pain in older adults with mild to moderate dementia. When severe dementia is present we need to consider alternative methods of assessment.

In the same literature review cited previously (20), 11 pain assessment tools were identified that are based upon pain behaviours. Although promising, these behavioural tools need to be evaluated more before they can be applied across the board.

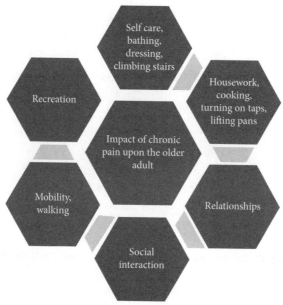

Fig. 12.1 Factors influencing chronic pain in the older adult.

The national pain assessment guidelines published in 2007 produced an algorithm which has been incorporated into an Android/iPhone application. This gives a decision pathway for pain assessment in older adults. It can be downloaded from <https://play.google.com/store/apps/details?id=com.gwizards. gre.ac.uk&feature=search_result#?t=W251bGwsMSwxLDEsImNvbS5nd2l6Y XJkcy5ncmUuYWMudWsiXQ> (22).

Whichever scale we use, it is important that we remember it may not just be the pain that is the problem for the older adult: it may also be factors that are impacted by the pain. Such factors include those in Figure 12.1.

The assessment guidelines recognize the need for a holistic, person-centred assessment; they also recognize that treatment may benefit from pharmacological and non-pharmacological methods of pain control. The World Health Organization's (23) three-step analgesic ladder is widely used for this purpose. Originally published in 1989, the ladder has been republished in 1996 and 2006.

7 Management of pain in the older population

For acute pain, analgesic management is the first-line approach with any group regardless of age. This is guided by the three-step ladder that has recently been reviewed and remains relevant today (24). (However, there is some controversy regarding the usefulness of the second step of the ladder.) The ladder provides a stepped approach and can be applied for the full range of pain from mild to severe:

- Step One: mild pain—simple analgesics; e.g. paracetamol and non-steroidal anti-inflammatory drugs (NSAIDs)

- Step Two: moderate pain—weak opioids; e.g. tramadol, codeine

- Step Three: severe pain—strong opioids; e.g. morphine, fentanyl, oxyco-done, pethidine.

Also relevant in this context are adjuvant analgesics: a group of drugs that were not originally developed to treat pain, but have been found to be useful for particular pain types, such as amitriptyline for neuropathic pain.

Of course, as discussed earlier, prescribing analgesic drugs for the older adult does need to take into consideration co-morbidities and potential for compromised systems, such as renal and hepatic metabolisms, which can affect the use of many drugs for pain relief. Also, there are many fears and worries that exist among health care professionals in terms of the use of strong opiate drugs. There have been a number of reviews of pharmacological management of persistent pain in older adults (25). 'Guidance on the Management of Pain in Older People' (26) is the first comprehensive pain guidance produced in the UK. It recommends management approaches that include pharmacological and non-pharmacological interventions. The guidance is summarized in Box 12.1.

In summary, paracetamol is the most appropriate drug for older adults, keeping in mind that dose reduction is necessary for frailer people. Opioid drugs are appropriate, but we should start low, go slowly, and acknowledge the risk of side effects. By anticipating such effects we can treat them before they occur. Adverse effects limit the use of the tricyclics in this population; routine monitoring of gastrointestinal, renal, and cardiovascular effects should be carried out when using NSAIDs. A co-prescription of a proton-pump inhibitor should be given.

Intra-articular corticosteroid injections in osteoarthritis of the knee are effective in relieving pain in the short term with little risk of complications, joint damage, or both. Intra-articular hyaluronic acid is effective and free of systemic adverse effects. It should be considered in patients intolerant to systemic therapy. Intra-articular hyaluronic acid appears to have a slower onset of action than intra-articular steroids, but the effects seem to last longer.

The current evidence for the use of epidural steroid injections in the management of sciatica is conflicting, and until larger studies become available, no firm recommendations can be made. There is, however, a limited body of evidence to support the use of epidural injections in spinal stenosis.

Assistive devices are widely used and ownership increases with age. Such devices enable older people with chronic pain to live in the community, but do not necessarily reduce pain and can even increase it if used incorrectly. Increasing activity by way of exercise should be considered and should involve

Box 12.1 'The Management of Pain in Older People' guidance summary

- Paracetamol should be considered as first-line treatment for the management of both acute and persistent pain, particularly of musculoskeletal origin, due to demonstrated efficacy and good safety profile.

- There are few absolute contraindications and relative cautions to prescribing paracetamol. It is important that the maximum daily dose (4 g/24 hours) is not exceeded and that dose is reduced for older adults under 50 kg.

- Non-steroidal anti-inflammatory drugs (NSAIDs) should be used with caution in older people after other safer treatments have not provided sufficient pain relief. The lowest dose should be provided for shortest duration.

- For older adults an NSAID or cyclo-oxygenase-2 selective inhibitor should be co-prescribed with a proton-pump inhibitor, choosing the one with the lowest acquisition cost.

- All older people taking NSAIDs should be routinely monitored for gastrointestinal, renal, and cardiovascular side effects, and drug–drug and drug–concomitant disease interactions.

- All patients with moderate and severe pain should be considered for opioid therapy, particularly if pain is causing functional impairment or reducing quality of life; however this must be individualized and carefully monitored.

- Opioid side effects, including nausea and vomiting, should be anticipated and suitable prophylaxis considered.

- Appropriate laxative therapy, such as the combination of a stool softener and a stimulant laxative, should be prescribed throughout treatment for all older people prescribed opioid therapy.

- Tricyclic antidepressants and anti-epileptic drugs have demonstrated efficacy in several types of neuropathic pain, but tolerability and adverse effects limit their use in an older population.

strengthening, flexibility, endurance, and balance along with a programme of education. Patient preference should be given serious consideration.

A number of complementary therapies have been found to have some efficacy among the older population, including acupuncture, TENS, and massage. Such approaches can affect pain and anxiety and are worth further investigation.

Some psychological approaches have been found to be useful for the older population as well, including guided imagery, biofeedback training, and relaxation. There is also some evidence supporting the use of cognitive behavioural therapy among nursing home populations, but of course these approaches require training and time.

In summary, both the American Geriatric Society guidelines and the British Pain Society/British Geriatric Society guidelines strongly recommend the use of paracetamol for the management of persistent pain. However, when the pain is acute and severe, paracetamol is often not enough. Poorly controlled acute pain can lead to delirium among this group, which can in turn lead to extended hospital stay or, even worse, long-term dependency upon health care (27). The alternative approach is to utilize opioids. Opioids however can have devastating effects upon the older adult: vomiting, constipation, respiratory depression, and sedation. These can impact mobility and ultimately delay recovery from surgery or injury. The general rule here is to avoid drugs such as pethidine completely as well as tramadol, which can cause nightmares in this population. Instead opt for the traditional approaches such as morphine, while using the approach of 'start low and go slow'.

8 Conclusion and future directions

An extensive search of the literature unearths very few publications specifically related to pain management the older adult. As discussed elsewhere in this book (Chapter 16), most of the research has been conducted in the younger population and extrapolated to older people. There is a clear need for further pain research for this group. Some ideas of future directions are given in Box 12.2.

Effective management of pain in the older person is limited by our lack of knowledge. The assumption that older adults 'get used to' or 'learn to live with' pain are unfounded. There is a plethora of effective pain assessment scales and an arsenal of pain management approaches for both acute and chronic pain. There is no need to develop more pain assessment tools for the older population; there is however an obligation to prevent unnecessary suffering due to reluctance to prescribe and administer effective pain relief. The Royal College of Surgeons stated that failure to relieve pain is morally and ethically unacceptable: adults are entitled to the best care that can be offered regardless of age (17). As the computer- and NHS-based generation gets older, expectations of pain-free surgery will increase. More demands will be placed upon the NHS to provide this care. Health care staff must be in the best position to assess and manage pain effectively; this will require better awareness of the latest pain assessment and management approaches. Should older adults be expected to live with

Box 12.2 Future directions?

+ Pain assessment should become a national standard for all areas where older adults are cared for.

+ There should be a national programme of evaluation looking at specific behavioural pain assessment tools and their application to practice to determine the most appropriate tool for use with adults with dementia.

+ More research needs to be developed looking at specific drugs and invasive interventions to determine the best approaches for pain management.

+ More research is needed into self-management techniques and complementary therapies and their impact upon pain in the older population.

+ We should consider ways of delivery of interventions such as new technologies, as well as their acceptability and feasibility.

pain? Is it a natural part of ageing? The answer is 'no'. There is a need for more research into pain assessment and management with this group, along with investigating ways of delivery to address a changing ageing population and the potential for isolation that occurs with remote and rural populations.

Websites and guidelines relevant to this chapter

National Service Framework for Older people—sets out the government's quality standards for health and social care services for older people:

<https://www.gov.uk/government/publications/quality-standards-for-care-services-for-older-people>

The British Pain Society—offers expert advice and guidance on all aspects of pain including specific guidance for the care of older adults in pain:

<http://www.britishpainsociety.org/>

The British Geriatric Society—offers guidance on all aspects of care for the older population including specific pain guidance:

<http://www.bgs.org.uk/>

References

1 D'Agostino NS, Gray G, Scanlon C. Cancer in the older adult: understanding age related changes. J Gerontol Nurs. 1990;**16**:12–15.

2 Bernabei R, Gambassi G, Lapane K, et al. Management of pain in elderly patients with cancer. SAGE (Systematic Assessment of Geriatric drug use via Epidemiology) Study Group. JAMA-J Am Med Assoc. 1998;**279**(23):1877–82.

3 **Schofield PA.** The assessment and management of peri-operative pain in older adults. Anaesthesia. 2014 Jan;**69**(suppl 1):54–60.

4 **Merskey H, Bogduk N.** Taxonomy of pain terms and definitions. Seattle: IASP Press; 1992.

5 **Desbiens NA, Mueller-Rizner N, Connors AF Jr, et al.** Pain in the oldest-old during hospitalization and up to one year later. J Am Geriatr Soc. 1997; **45**:1167–72.

6 **Catananti C, Gambassi G.** Pain assessment in the elderly. Surg Oncol. 2010;**19**(3):140–8.

7 **Aubrun F.** French Society of Anesthesia and Resuscitation. Ann Fr Anesth Reanim. 2009 Jan;**28**(1):e39–41.

8 **Harkins SW, Davis MD, Bush FM, Kasberger J.** Suppression of first pain and slow temporal summation of second pain in relation to age. J Gerontol A-Biol. 1996;**51A**:M260–M26.

9 **Egbert AM.** Postoperative pain management in the frail elderly. Clin Geriatr Med. 1996 Aug;**12**(3):583–99.

10 **Epstein JB, Schubert MM.** Oral mucositis in myelosuppressive cancer therapy. Oral Surg Oral Med Oral Pathol Oral Radiol Endod. 1999;**88**:273–6.

11 **Eisenach JC, Curry R, Tong C, Houle TT, Yaksh TL.** Effects of intrathecal ketorolac on human experimental pain Anesthesiology. Author manuscript; available in PMC 2011 May 1. Anesthesiology. 2010 May;**112**(5):1216–24.

12 **Gibson SJ, Farrell M.** A review of age differences in the neurophysiology of nociception and the perceptual experience of pain. Clin J Pain. 2004 Jul-Aug;**20**(4):227–39.

13 **Helme RD.** How useful are currently available tools for pain evaluation in elderly people with dementia? Nat Clin Pract Neurol. 2006 Sep;**2**(9):474–5.

14 **Farrell MJ.** Age-related changes in the structure and function of brain regions involved in pain processing. Pain Med. 2012 Apr;**13** Suppl 2:S37–43.

15 **Conway V, Schofield PA.** 2013. Pain assessment in nursing homes in one county. Presentation at the British Geriatric Society, Belfast.

16 **Ahn H, Horgas A.** The relationship between pain and disruptive behaviors in nursing home residents with dementia. BMC Geriatr. 2013;**13**:14. Epub 2013 Feb 11. doi: 10.1186/1471-2318-134

17 **Royal College of Surgeons, College of Anaesthetists.** Pain after surgery. Sep 1990. Accessed 16 Jun 2014. http://www.rcoa.ac.uk/system/files/FPM-Pain-After-Surgery.pdf

18 **Joint Commission on Accreditation of Healthcare Organizations.** Implementing the new pain management standards. Oakbrook Terrace, IL: JCAHO; 2000

19 **Schofield P, O'Mahony S, Collett B, Potter J.** Guidance for the assessment of pain in older adults: a literature review. Br J Nurs. 2008 Jul 24–Aug 13;**17**(14):914–8.

20 **Herr K, Bjoro K, Decker S.** Tools for assessment of pain in nonverbal older adults with dementia: a state-of-the-science review. Journal of Pain and Symptom Management. 2006 Feb;**31**(2):170–192.

21 **British Geriatrics Society/British Pain Society.** Guidelines for the assessment of pain in older adults. 2007. Accessed 16 Jun 2014. http://www.bgs.org.uk/index.php/clinicalguides/313-painassessment

22 **University of Greenwich pain assessment application.** http://www.youtube.com/watch?v=3hv5WJEtflA or https://itunes.apple.com/WebObjects/MZStore.woa/wa/viewSoftware?id=669494624&mt=8

23 **The WHO Pain Ladder**. http://www.who.int/cancer/palliative/painladder/en/ Accessed 9 Oct 2013.

24 **Vargas-Schaffer G**. Is the WHO analgesic ladder still valid? Twenty-four years of experience. Can Fam Physician. 2010 Jun;**56**(6):514–7.

25 **American Geriatric Society**. Management of persistent pain in older adults. Accessed 9 Oct 2013. http://www.americangeriatrics.org/health_care_professionals/clinical_practice/clinical_guidelines_recommendations/2009/

26 **Abdulla A, et al**. Guidance on the management of pain in older people. Age Ageing. 2013 Mar;42(suppl 1):i1–57.

27 **Abou-Setta AM, Beaupre LA, Rashiq S, Dryden DM, Hamm MP, Sadowski CA, Menon MR, Majumdar SR, Wilson DM, Karkhaneh M, Mousavi SS, Wong K, Tjosvold L, Jones CA**. Comparative effectiveness of pain management interventions for hip fracture: a systematic review. Ann Intern Med. 2011 Aug 16;**155**(4):234–45. doi: 10.7326/0003–4819–155–4–201108160–0346

Chapter 13

Stroke units: research in practice

Lalit Kalra

Key points

- Stroke units are the cornerstone of quality stroke care.
- The benefits of stroke unit care are supported by a very strong evidence base
- In 2007 the National Stroke Strategy mandated that all stroke patients should have prompt access to stroke unit care.
- Despite policy and guidelines, only 62% stroke patients were treated on specialist stroke units in 2010.
- Patients spend long periods of inactivity on stroke units; multidisciplinary teams need to encourage rehabilitation activities outside therapy sessions.
- Rehabilitation needs to be family- and carer-oriented to prepare patients for life after discharge.

1 Introduction

Twenty years ago, stroke rehabilitation was given low priority by health care professionals and planners: it was considered to be at the periphery of health service provision. A Consensus Conference on Stroke was held in London in 1988 with invited experts. It concluded that services for stroke patients were haphazard, with no clear policy on planning or implementation (1). There was a striking lack of convincing evidence for widely used rehabilitative treatments and a serious shortage of treatment—patients were unoccupied for long periods. This picture of disorganized and ineffective care was further strengthened by outcome studies showing significant variations in case fatality and levels of independence after treatment across different areas of the country (2). The studies indicated poor performance on these measures when the UK was compared with other Western European and international centres (3).

In contrast, the National Stroke Strategy in 2007 (4) mandated that all stroke patients have prompt access to an acute stroke unit and spend the majority of their time at hospital in a stroke unit with high-quality stroke specialist care. This was based on overwhelming evidence that stroke units reduce death and increase the number of independent and non-institutionalized individuals, with proven benefits for five and ten years. An estimation of this benefit is provided by the National Sentinel Audit report, which calculated that if timely access to stroke units were increased to 75% of stroke patients, this would prevent more than 500 deaths per year and result in more than 200 more independent individuals (5).

The remarkable transition of stroke management from being in the shadows to its prominent position in UK health care today is testimony to the impact that research has on improving clinical care and patient outcomes. It is true that another major development—the introduction of thrombolysis for acute stroke patients in clinical practice—has revolutionized the management of stroke patients, but the trial benefits of thrombolysis do not translate equally into clinical effectiveness in mainstream practice (6). The proportion of patients with ischaemic stroke varies between settings, and the 4.5-hour time window for thrombolysis severely limits the benefits of an otherwise powerful intervention. Many studies have shown that only 25–33% of patients present to hospitals within thrombolysis time windows onset (7) and only a small proportion, 5–20%, of incident ischaemic stroke actually end up being thrombolyzed. Although National Stroke Audit data show that the thrombolysis rates rose from 1–2% to 5% of the stroke population with the implementation of the National Stroke Strategy, the majority of stroke patients remain excluded from the benefits of thrombolysis. In contrast, stroke units can benefit the vast majority of stroke patients regardless of pathology or time of presentation (8).

2 The rationale for stroke unit care

As early as the 1990s, research showed that organized care provided on stroke units facilitates neurological recovery and expedites discharges (Figure 13.1) (9). More recently, positron emission tomography (PET) and magnetic resonance imaging (MRI) studies have confirmed the concept of brain plasticity, which implies that it is possible to modulate or facilitate reorganization of cerebral processes by external inputs (10). The paradigm for function has shifted from strict cerebral localization to that of interactive functioning multiple motor circuits activated by the constantly changing balance of inhibitory and excitatory impulses. Disruption of major pathways in stroke reduces the inhibition normally exerted by these pathways and allows activation of alternate pathways,

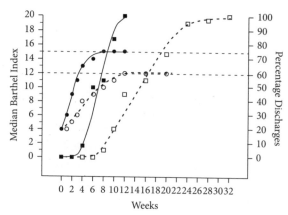

Fig. 13.1 The effect of stroke units on the speed and extent of functional recovery (Barthel Index) and weeks to discharge from inpatient settings (8).
A = Barthel Index of patients managed on the stroke rehabilitation unit (●, ■)
B = Barthel Index of patients managed on general medical wards (○, □)
A vs B, $p = 0.001$

which take over the function of the damaged circuits. Furthermore, neuroimaging studies have shown that increased intensity of therapy results in greater activation of areas associated with the function towards which therapy was directed (11). Hence, evidence suggests that the human brain is capable of significant recovery after stroke, provided that the appropriate treatments and stimuli are applied in adequate amounts and at the right time. It is likely that this is achieved better with organized stroke care, where the intensity and timing of interventions can be managed proactively.

Stroke affects several domains of human performance and results in multiple impairments, many of which interact to determine the level of disability. No single discipline has all the skills, resources, and expertise required to manage all impairments associated with stroke. Furthermore, different impairments recover at different speeds, requiring a staged approach to therapy interventions. Rehabilitation goals are also shaped by personal needs of stroke patients, the environment they will return to, and the personal support available after discharge. Hence, the complex interdisciplinary process of stroke rehabilitation requires a multidisciplinary approach and collaborative policy of coordinated delivery of treatments. Such treatments need to be based on comprehensive assessments and delivered by staff trained in stroke management, in consultation with patients and their caregivers. This level of coordination of care is another argument in support of specialist stroke units (12).

3 The evidence for stroke unit care

In the 1980s and 1990s, a number of randomized controlled trials suggested that organized care offers advantages to patients with stroke. However, many of these studies were too small to demonstrate a robust statistical benefit. Studies were also undertaken in different settings, using different methods of organized care, and using stroke patients at varying duration from stroke onset. Interventions ranged from acute dedicated units to teams providing coordinated care in community settings; the patients ranged from those within a few hours of stroke onset to those included only when they were neurologically and medically stable. In order to obtain meaningful evidence relevant to clinical practice, the Stroke Unit Trialists' Collaboration (SUTC) pooled data from all studies that met strict inclusion and quality-control criteria from different centres. The meta-analysis of pooled data from 29 trials, which include 6,536 patients, shows odds reductions in mortality of 0.86 (95% CI: 0.71–0.94), death or dependence of 0.78 (95% CI: 0.68–0.89), and death or institution of 0.80 (95% CI: 0.71–0.90) at one year are associated with organized care, independent of age and gender (13). More important, and in contrast with thrombolysis for acute stroke, these benefits are seen for all stroke patients regardless of stroke aetiology or the duration between stroke onset and intervention. Furthermore, the translation of trial efficacy outcomes into clinical effectiveness in mainstream practice has been demonstrated in longitudinal studies (14).

4 Processes that contribute to a good outcome

Organized stroke unit care is considered a 'black box' intervention: there is no one single process of care or intervention that has been shown to be responsible for better outcomes. A major problem in the generalizability of different interventions or processes of care is that most stroke units have evolved in response to local patient needs, priorities, and service arrangements, which may not be replicated in other settings (15). Hence, the same process may have a different impact on outcomes on different units, depending upon case mix, the type of unit, and the environment in which the unit functions. Survival is strongly associated, however, with processes of care that are carried out significantly more frequently on stroke units. These include comprehensive and early stroke-specific assessments, particularly assessments for swallowing and aspiration risk, early detection and management of infections, maintenance of hydration and nutrition, early mobilization, clear goals for function, and communication with patients and their families (16). In addition to doctors and nurses, speech and language therapists, physiotherapists, occupational therapists, and dieticians have specific contributions to make in delivering these particular aspects of care. The probable explanation for higher survival and lower institutionalization rates on stroke units are attributable to improved medical management, prevention of complications, and coordination of multidisciplinary care.

5 Issues in providing stroke unit care

Although evidence strongly supports stroke units for reducing mortality, dependence, and institutionalization in stroke patients, the benefits expected from stroke units are not fully realized in day-to-day clinical practice. The National Stroke Audit in 2000 showed that only 18% of patients were managed on a stroke unit for the majority of their stay. By 2010 this rose to 62%, but it still implies that more than one in three patients are denied stroke unit care. In England the number of hospitals with a stroke unit increased from 40% to 98% between 2000 and 2010, but—despite all the investments made into stroke care—there are still disparities in stroke outcome between centres in the UK. Very often, poor outcomes are attributed to the lack of investment, but comparisons show that the UK spends more than most of its European neighbours on stroke care, especially on specialist stroke services (17). Possible explanations include differences between what has been recommended and what actually has been implemented in the organization of stroke services, compliance of the staff with multidisciplinary guidelines, variations in how multidisciplinary teams function, and the tailoring of rehabilitation to the priorities of stroke patients and their caregivers.

5.1 **Organization of stroke units**

There is considerable debate about what constitutes a stroke unit (18). Definitions vary from 'a team of specialists who are knowledgeable about the care of stroke patients and who consult throughout a hospital or the community wherever a patient may be' to 'a geographic location within the hospital designated for stroke and stroke-like patients who are in need of medical and rehabilitation services and the skilled professional care that such an unit can provide.' There is also considerable controversy on the number and diversity of disciplines that need to be involved in stroke care. Differences in staff composition between different settings have limited the generalization of findings in individual settings. The prevalent strategies for providing specialist stroke care are summarized in Table 13.1. Langhorne et al. (19) have shown that there is a definite benefit associated with comprehensive and rehabilitation stroke units and mixed rehabilitation units, all of which show an odds ratio of 0.85 to 0.89 in favour of organized care. There is also a possible benefit with acute (semi-intensive) units, although this just fails to achieve statistical significance (OR 0.88; 95% CI: 0.76–1.01).

Table 13.1 Different types of stroke care organization (17)

Type	Admission	Discharge	Features
Acute, intensive	Acute (hours)	Days	High nurse staffing Life support facilities
Acute, semi-intensive	Acute (hours)	Days	Close physiological monitoring
Comprehensive	Acute (hours)	Days–weeks	Acute care/rehabilitation Conventional staffing
Rehabilitation	Delayed	Weeks	Rehabilitation
Mobile team	Variable	Days–weeks	Medical/rehabilitation advice
Mixed rehabilitation	Variable	Weeks	Mixed patient group Rehabilitation

Mobile stroke teams were associated with no benefit in this analysis (OR 0.98; 95% CI: 0.95–1.05). There are no trials of acute intensive care.

In 2005, 40% hospitals had a stroke unit but less than half of them met the criteria of stroke unit, and more than a quarter did not meet even the basic standards for rehabilitation care (20). The situation has changed since then. The 2010 National Audit showed that 98% hospitals in the UK have a stroke unit and approximately 60% of stroke patients actually received care for the majority of their hospital stay on such units.

5.2 Multidisciplinary practice on stroke units

Comprehensive multidisciplinary guidelines for stroke unit care have been available across the UK for several years, but recommended standards are met in only 25–60% of patients treated in specialist settings (21). This is because several professional therapist societies have their own sets of standards, which are different enough from those recommended by the Multidisciplinary Stroke Guideline Working Group to affect practice. There are limited opportunities for multidisciplinary education or training on many units; implementation is further hampered by the experience, personal preferences, and established practices of individuals within the stroke unit. Furthermore, many of the expected advantages of multidisciplinary teamwork are influenced by composition, location, and interactions between various team members. Contrary to the popularly held view that multidisciplinary teams improve care, a study has also shown that teamwork in rehabilitation settings resulted in lack of professional accountability or personal responsibility among team members and reduced patient contact time (22). The Collaborative Evaluation of Rehabilitation In Stroke across Europe (CERISE) study compared stroke rehabilitation units across four settings in Europe. It showed that patients in UK stroke units spent nearly 65% of the working day sitting, lying, or sleeping and had greater contact with visitors than with therapists. Compared with other centres, stroke units in the UK committed the greatest amount of therapy resources (70 hours/week); nevertheless, stroke patients in the UK received the least amount of therapy input (1 hour/day). The discrepancy is explained by the fact that most of therapy time in the UK was spent on administrative and non-therapeutic activities (23).

5.3 The effect of stroke severity on benefits from organized care

A limitation of most randomized controlled studies on organized care is that they included patients with moderate stroke severity and excluded those with mild or very severe strokes. An analysis of pooled RCT data for patients stratified according to stroke severity at the time of inclusion showed that organized stroke care prevented 1 death/100 patients in patients with mild stroke (Barthel Index 10–20), 3 deaths/100 patients in the those with moderate stroke (Barthel Index 3–9), and 9 deaths/100 patients in those with severe stroke (Barthel Index 0–2) (24). This suggests that the benefits of organized inpatient care for mortality increase with stroke severity; that is, the absolute reduction in deaths is greater for patients with more severe stroke. The analysis also showed that most of the deaths prevented were those that would have occurred at one to four weeks after stroke onset and would be attributable to stroke-related complications. The heterogeneity in data prevented the assessment of the interaction between organized stroke care and functional recovery, which would be particularly important for patients with mild stroke, where organized care, understandably, has no effect on mortality.

5.4 Involving patients and caregivers

Very often, in open-ended health care systems such as the NHS, the duration of rehabilitation of patients has been unnecessarily prolonged because the rehabilitation goals of professionals do not reflect the recovery priorities of patients or their caregivers. The importance of matching professional and patient priorities for improving the effectiveness and efficiency of stroke rehabilitation is becoming increasingly evident in the qualitative stroke literature (25). Patients define recovery in relation to their own social context and their own expectations from rehabilitation, whereas professionals measure recovery in terms of actual gains in function against those expected for the severity of impairment. Furthermore, the goals of patients are often seen as subordinate to those of professionals. Unrealistic anticipation of the degree of recovery by patients is not managed adequately, resulting in delayed or contested discharges from inpatient settings. Despite the proven effectiveness of rehabilitation in outpatient and community settings (26), there is often a reluctance, quite often justified, in patients to leave the certainty of inpatient therapy for uncertain rehabilitation in the community (27).

Although the physical, psychological, emotional, and social consequences of caregiving and its economic benefit to society are well-recognized, caregivers' needs are often given low priority in stroke management. Many caregivers feel inadequately trained, poorly informed, and dissatisfied with level of support after discharge (28). An important challenge for stroke units is a conceptual shift in the philosophy of stroke care from being predominantly engaged with patient-oriented interventions to a strategy in which the patient and the caregiver are seen as a combined focus for intervention. The objective should be to empower and equip caregivers to be competent facilitators of activities of daily living when caring for disabled stroke patients (29).

6 Future challenges for stroke units

Organized stroke care, such as that provided by stroke units, improves outcomes for patients regardless of stroke severity, but those with more severe strokes have more to gain from such management. Despite the advances made in organized stroke care in the last decade, there remains considerable scope for improvement and continued evolution in response to patient and caregiver needs, new therapies, and the changing environment of health care provision.

It is of concern that despite most hospitals in the UK having stroke units, a significant proportion of stroke patients do not receive stroke unit care for the whole or a part of their stay in hospital. Furthermore, stroke sentinel audits continue to show that there is a great disparity in the quality of care that patients receive between units, even ones with comparable resources. The first challenge, then, must be to ensure that all stroke patients spend the vast majority of their time in specialist settings and that the best quality of care is received by all patients, regardless of the stroke unit on which they are managed. This has been addressed in the latest guidelines from the National Institute of Health and Clinical Excellence and the Royal College of Physicians (see suggested websites at the end of this chapter).

Studies have shown that patients on stroke units spend more than 50% time of their in bed, 28% sitting out of bed, and only 13% in therapeutic activities. Indeed they are alone for 60% of the therapeutic day (30). The second challenge, therefore, is to develop strategies that increase the intensity of therapeutic activities and interaction with patients.

It is estimated that 25–74% of stroke survivors require assistance with activities for daily living from informal caregivers, often family members. The needs of caregivers are poorly recognized and managed on stroke units; the third challenge then must be to empower and equip caregivers for their new role.

7 **Conclusion**

Stroke units are central to providing high-quality stroke care both for acute management and rehabilitation. The effectiveness of stroke units in improving patient outcomes and reducing costs of care are supported by strong research evidence. Unlike other interventions, stroke units can benefit almost all stroke patients regardless of age, sex, stroke severity, and delays in presentation to hospital. Based on the strength of evidence, the National Stroke Strategy mandated that all stroke patients should have prompt access to stroke unit care. In response to policy changes, the number of hospitals with stroke units in England increased from 40% to 98% between 2000 and 2010, and the number of patients receiving care on these units for the majority of stay rose from 18% to 62%.

Despite these improvements, several challenges remain in stroke care. Recent studies have challenged the effectiveness of the way in which multidisciplinary care is delivered and there is a need for further exploration on improving this care. Similarly studies have shown that most stroke patients on specialist units spend large periods with no activities. The challenge for multidisciplinary teams is to fill this time with therapeutic rehabilitation activities. Finally, research has shown that training of carers is an important element for ensuring smooth transition to life at home following hospital discharge. The focus of rehabilitation needs to move from being patient-oriented to being patient-and-carer-oriented.

Websites relevant to this chapter

National Stroke Audit 2010—reports performance against quality benchmarks for stroke units in England and Wales:

<http://www.rcplondon.ac.uk/sites/default/files/sentinel_public_clinical_report_2010.pdf>

National Stroke Strategy—sets the standards of care for stroke patients:

<http://www.dh.gov.uk/prod_consum_dh/groups/dh_digitalassets/documents/digitalasset/dh_081059.pdf>

Stroke Care Pathways—describe the recommended management of stroke patients during the acute and rehabilitation phases of their care:

<http://pathways.nice.org.uk/pathways/stroke#path=view%3A/pathways/stroke/acute-stroke.xml&content=close>

<http://pathways.nice.org.uk/pathways/stroke#path=view%3A/pathways/stroke/stroke-rehabilitation.xml&content=close>

Clinical Guideline for Stroke Unit Care—quality standards and guidelines for the management of stroke patients from stroke onset to aftercare in the community:

<http://guidance.nice.org.uk/CG68>

<http://guidance.nice.org.uk/CG162>

<http://www.rcplondon.ac.uk/sites/default/files/national-clinical-guidelines-for-stroke-fourth-edition.pdf>

Key guidelines, policy documents, and reviews

Meta-analysis of trials of stroke unit care: Stroke Unit Trialists Collaboration. Organized inpatient (stroke unit) care for stroke (31).

Components of stroke unit care: Langhorne P, Pollock A. What are the components of effective stroke unit care? (32).

Key guidelines on stroke rehabilitation (NICE, 2012):

<http://guidance.nice.org.uk/CG162>

Meta-analysis of trials of comprehensive geriatric assessment:

Ellis et al. (33) Comprehensive geriatric assessment for older adults admitted to hospital.

References

1 **Consensus conference.** Treatment of stroke. BMJ. 1988 Jul 9;**297**(6641): 126–8.

2 **Rudd AG, Irwin P, Rutledge Z, Lowe D, Wade DT, Pearson M.** Royal College of Physicians Intercollegiate Stroke Working Party. Regional variations in stroke care in England, Wales and Northern Ireland: results from the National Sentinel Audit of Stroke. Clin Rehabil. 2001 Oct;**15**(5):562–72.

3 **Weir NU, Sandercock PA, Lewis SC, Signorini DF, Warlow CP.** Variations between countries in outcome after stroke in the International Stroke Trial (IST). Stroke. 2001 Jun;**32**(6):1370–7.

4 **Department of Health.** National Stroke Strategy, 2007. London: HMSO.

5 **Royal College of Physicians,** Clinical Effectiveness and Evaluation Unit. National Sentinel Stroke Audit 2006. Royal College of Physicians of London; 2007.

6 **Barber M, Langhorne P, Stott DJ.** Barriers to delivery of thrombolysis for acute stroke. Age Ageing. 2004 Mar;**33**(2):94–5.

7 **Harraf F, Sharma AK, Brown MM, Lees KR, Vass RI, Kalra L.** A multicentre observational study of presentation and early assessment of acute stroke. BMJ. 2002;**325**:17–21.

8 **Kalra L, Langhorne P.** Facilitating recovery: Evidence for organised stroke care. Journal of Rehabilitation 2007;**39**:97–102.

9 **Kalra L.** The influence of stroke unit rehabilitation on functional recovery from stroke. Stroke 1994;**25**(4):821–5.

10 Sztriha LK, O'Gorman RL, Modo M, Barker GJ, Williams SCR, Kalra L. Monitoring brain repair in stroke using advanced magnetic resonance imaging. Stroke. 2012 Nov;**43**(11):3124–31.

11 Johansen-Berg H, Dawes H, Guy C, Smith SM, Wade DT, Matthews PM. Correlation between motor improvements and altered fMRI activity after rehabilitative therapy. Brain. 2002;**125**(Pt 12):2731–42.

12 Langhorne P, Cadilhac D, Feigin V, Grieve R, Liu M. How should stroke services be organised? Lancet Neurol. 2002;**1**(1):62–8.

13 Stroke Unit Trialists' Collaboration. Organized inpatient (stroke unit) care for stroke. Cochrane Database Syst Rev. 2002;(**1**):CD000197.

14 Fjaertoft H, Indredavik B, Lydersen S. Stroke unit care combined with early supported discharge: long-term follow-up of a randomized controlled trial. Stroke. 2003;**34**(11):2687–91.

15 Indredavik B, Bakke F, Slordahl SA, Rokseth R, Haheim LL. Treatment in a combined acute and rehabilitation stroke unit: which aspects are most important? Stroke. 1999; **30**(5):917–23.

16 Evans A, Perez I, Harraf F, Melbourn M, Steadman J, Donaldson N, Kalra L. Can differences in management processes explain different outcomes between stroke unit and stroke team care? Lancet 2001;**358**:1586–92.

17 Epstein D, Mason A, Manca A. The hospital costs of care for stroke in nine European countries. Health Econ. 2008 Jan;**17**(1 Suppl):S21–31.

18 Stroke Unit Trialists Collaboration. Collaborative systemic review of the randomised trials of organised inpatient (Stroke Unit) care after stroke. BMJ 1997;**314**:1151–8.

19 Langhorne P for Stroke Unit Trialists Collaboration. The effect of different types of organized inpatient (stroke unit) care. Cerebrovasc Dis 2005;**19**(Suppl 2):68.

20 Rudd AG, Hoffman A, Irwin P, Pearson M, Lowe D. Stroke units: research and reality. Results from the National Sentinel Audit of Stroke. Qual Saf Health Care 2005;**14**;7–12.

21 Hammond R, Lennon S, Walker MF, Hoffman A, Irwin P, Lowe D. Changing occupational therapy and physiotherapy practice through guidelines and audit in the United Kingdom. Clin Rehab 2005;**19**:365.

22 Baxter SK, Brumfitt SM. Benefits and losses: a qualitative study exploring healthcare staff perceptions of teamworking. J Eval Clin Pract 2008;**17**:127–30.

23 De Wit L, Putman K, Schuback B, Komarek A, Angst F, Baert I, Berman P, et al. Motor and functional recovery after stroke: a comparison of 4 European rehabilitation centers. Stroke 2007;**38**:2101–7.

24 Langhorne P for Stroke Unit Trialists Collaboration. The effect of organized inpatient (stroke unit) care on death after stroke. Cerebrovasc Dis. 2005;**19**(Suppl 2):68.

25 McKevitt C, Redfern J, Mold F, Wolfe C. Qualitative studies of stroke—a systematic review. Stroke. 2004;**35**:1499–1505.

26 Aziz NA, Leonardi-Bee J, Phillips M, Gladman JR, Legg L, Walker MF. Therapy-based rehabilitation services for patients living at home more than one year after stroke. Cochrane Database Syst Rev. 2008 Apr;**16**(2):CD005952.

27 Mold F, Wolfe C, McKevitt C. Falling through the net of stroke care. Health Soc Care Community. 2006 Jul;**14**(4):349–56.

28 Kalra L, Evans A, Perez I, Melbourn A, Patel A, Knapp M, Donaldson N. Training care givers of stroke patients: Randomised controlled trial. BMJ. 2004;**328**(7448):1099–1101.

29 **McCullagh E, Brigstocke G, Donaldson N, Kalra L**. Determinants of caregiving burden and quality of life in caregivers of stroke patients Stroke 2005;**36**(10): 2181–6.

30 **Bernhardt J, Dewey H, Thrift A, Donnan G**. Inactive and alone: physical activity within the first 14 days of acute stroke unit care. Stroke. 2004;**35**(4):1005–9.

31 **Stroke Unit Trialists Collaboration**. Organized inpatient (stroke unit) care for stroke. Cochrane Database Syst Rev. 2009;CD000197. http://onlinelibrary.wiley.com/doi/10.1002/14651858.CD000197.pub2/pdf

32 **Langhorne P, Pollock A**. Stroke Unit Trialists' Collaboration. What are the components of effective stroke unit care? Age Ageing. 2002 Sep;**31**(5):365–71.

33 **Ellis G, Whitehead MA, Robinson D, O'Neill D, Langhorne P**. Comprehensive geriatric assessment for older adults admitted to hospital: meta-analysis of randomised controlled trials. BMJ. 2011;**343**:d6553.

Chapter 14

Stroke care: what is in the black box?

Christine Roffe

Key points

- Most improvements in stroke care to date have been driven by research.
- Immediate access to advanced imaging allows fast decision making, is cost-effective, and improves outcome.
- Hyperacute interventions for acute ischaemic and haemorrhagic stroke can prevent permanent brain damage and reduce disability.
- Strokes and stroke complications do not just happen during working hours: 24/7 working is essential for effective stroke management.
- High quality nursing care is essential and has been shown to have a major impact on survival.
- Pneumonia is the most common post-stroke complication, and can be prevented by early swallow assessment.
- Urinary catheters are associated with infections and should be avoided.
- Foot pumps reduce thromboembolism and save lives.

1 Introduction

It is well established that stroke units save lives, reduce disability, and allow more stroke survivors to return to their own homes (1). Evidence suggesting a benefit from treatment in dedicated stroke units first emerged in the 1980s with single unit trials, but has only been widely accepted after statistical significance of the survival advantage for patients treated in stroke units was shown in a systematic review (2). It has nevertheless been argued that stroke units tested in RCTs are not representative and that benefits may be overestimated (3). This concern has been put to rest by a recent review of observational studies of stroke units in their natural habitat which showed that the benefit associated with stroke-unit care in routine clinical practice is comparable to that seen in RCTs (4). Furthermore, evidence is now emerging that benefit from stroke-unit care is not restricted to the largely Anglo-American and Scandinavian 'homelands' of stroke-unit trials, but can also be shown in other health care systems throughout the world (5, 6). What is less clear is which aspects of organized stroke care determine better outcome.

Evidence for stroke-unit care, different types of stroke unit, which patients benefit, and current practice is reviewed by Kalra (Chapter 13). The aims of this chapter will be to describe key aspects of the content of the stroke unit 'black box' and how various interventions have been shaped by evidence or the lack thereof. The chapter will end with a brief exploration of future developments in stroke care and research.

2 Structural elements of specialist stroke services

Stroke units in the UK can be classified either by the stage of stroke recovery of the patient: hyperacute (the first 72 h after stroke), acute, rehabilitation, and combined units, or by the services that the unit provides: comprehensive stroke centres, primary stroke centres, and acute stroke-ready hospitals. The US Brain Attack Coalition defines a comprehensive stroke centre as a facility that provides high-intensity medical and surgical care, specialized diagnostics, and interventional therapies (7). Key elements of primary stroke centres include acute stroke teams, stroke units, written care protocols, an integrated emergency response system, availability and interpretation of computed tomography scans 24 hours a day, rapid laboratory testing, administrative support, strong leadership, and continuing education (8). In 2011 the coalition authors refined the recommendations (9) into seven key requirements:

◆ acute stroke teams

◆ telemetry monitoring

◆ brain imaging with MRI

◆ assessment of cerebral vasculature with magnetic resonance (MR) or computerized tomography (CT) angiography

◆ cardiac imaging

◆ early initiation of rehabilitation

◆ certification by an independent body, including site visits and disease performance measures.

A third type of facility, the acute stroke-ready hospital, has fewer capabilities and more limited resources, but is organized to diagnose, stabilize, treat, and transfer most patients with stroke. In 2013 the European Stroke Organization published criteria for stroke units and stroke centres. These specify 37 and 65 requirements for certification of the two types of unit respectively, and cover, inter alia, departments, staff, facilities for investigation, hyperacute interventions, protocols, pathways, monitoring, assessment, and multiprofessional teams (10). In the UK requirements for stroke units are summarized in the National Stroke Guidelines published by the Royal College of Physicians (2012), with more detail in the Stroke Service Standards (11) and the Consultant Workforce Requirements (12) by the British Association of Stroke Physicians.

While new acute interventions such as thrombolysis and endovascular treatments for stroke emphasize the need for hyperacute or comprehensive stroke centres, the strongest evidence for the effectiveness of stroke units is based on trials conducted later in the stroke journey in combined and rehabilitation stroke units (13), and relates to interventions aimed at prevention of complications rather than the brain injury.

3 Key aspects of stroke-unit practice and treatment associated with good outcome

3.1 Hyperacute stroke treatments

Over the past two decades a number of acute stroke treatments have been developed and shown to be effective in clinical trials. This research has changed the face of stroke care and introduced the concept of stroke medicine. Ischaemic stroke is caused by blockage of an artery supplying part of the brain, causing cell death and loss of function. The key concept underlying hyperacute stroke care is that symptoms can be reversed and the stroke aborted or reduced in severity if this artery can be unblocked before cell death occurs. Thrombolysis with alteplase was first shown to be effective for patients under the age of 80 years if given within three hours of symptom onset by the National Institutes of Neurological Disorders stroke trial in 1995 (14). The time frame was subsequently extended to 4.5 h with the results of the ECASS-3 trial (15), and inclusion widened to patients over the age of 80 following the IST-3 study (16). The results of IST-3 also confirm that 'time is brain', with the potential for full recovery highest when treatment is started within 90 minutes, and little or no benefit after 4.5 hours.

Intravenous thrombolysis is contraindicated in patients with increased bleeding risk. Timely recanalization with intravenous thrombolysis is considerably less likely if the thrombus burden is large, such as in occlusions of the carotid, proximal middle cerebral, and basilar arteries. Mechanical thrombectomy, using a device introduced via the femoral artery into the occluded brain vessel to extract the clot, can be used where thrombolysis is contraindicated or has failed. A systematic review of case series suggests that this can be performed safely (mean mortality 17%, range 4–44%) and is at least as effective, if not more so, than intravenous thrombolysis (independent recovery in 42%, range 15–54%) (17). The first RCTs of intra-arterial thrombolysis and/or thrombectomy (IMS-3, MRRESCUE, SYNTHESIS) have not shown significant benefits over conventional treatment. Those studies, however, had significant limitations: outdated devices, low treatment rate, and very late interventions (18). Several studies using newer devices and tighter inclusion criteria are ongoing (MRCLEAN, THRACE, PISTE).

Decompressive hemicraniectomy significantly improves survival in young patients with a large ischaemic stroke and malignant middle cerebral oedema, previously an almost invariably fatal condition. The number of patients who need to be treated with this procedure to save one life (NNT) is as low as two (19). More recently decompressive hemicraniectomy has also been shown to be effective in older people up to the age of 82 years with a NNT of 4 (20).

Arguably one of the most important reasons for recent improvements in stroke outcomes is the availability of acute and hyperacute treatments. While these are still applicable only to a very small proportion of stroke patients, the idea that something can be done has changed attitudes of medical staff from seeing stroke as a fate to be managed to a disease to be treated.

3.2 Better management of intracerebral haemorrhage

Stroke-unit care does not only benefit patients with cerebral infarcts. It also benefits those with intracerebral haemorrhage, with a 38% reduction in 30-day mortality ($p = 0.007$) (21). There is no robust evidence to support any specific therapeutic strategy, but there is good evidence that some interventions are not beneficial. These include the administration of corticosteroids (22), early surgery for intracerebral haemorrhage (23), and haemostatic therapy in patients with normal coagulation (22). Following common sense, but not formally tested, approaches such as rapid correction of coagulation disorders, control of very high blood pressure, stabilization of haemodynamic parameters, early mobilization to prevent thromboembolism, adequate nutrition, airway hygiene, and good nursing care are all likely to contribute to better outcomes.

The negative results of the STICH and STICH-2 (23, 24) trials comparing early surgery with delayed surgery are often falsely interpreted to mean that surgery for intracerebral haemorrhage is not effective. But patients were included only when the surgeon was uncertain about benefits of 'immediate' (e.g. within 12 hours) intervention. Neither trial addressed the question of effectiveness of surgery as such, but rather the timing of the intervention. In the management of cerebral infarct, 'early' relates to the first 4.5 hours after symptom onset, but in the STICH studies 'early' was defined as up to 60 hours after the ictus. This may have been too late for prevention of secondary brain damage. Nevertheless, both trials showed a non-significant reduction in death and disability. While this result does not give a clear indication for surgery, it definitely shows that patients were not harmed by early intervention. Surgery should therefore still be considered in selected patients fit for the procedure.

Potential indications for surgery are large cerebellar haemorrhages and cortical haematomas >30 ml and less than 1 cm from the surface (25). A trial of tight blood pressure control (INTERACT-2) with rapid reduction of the systolic pressure to 140 mmHg has also shown a trend towards better outcomes (26).

Conversely, early withdrawal of active management is associated with adverse outcomes. In particular, early institution of do-not- resuscitate (DNR) orders is associated with an increased risk of death, even after correction for case mix and co-morbidities. The American Heart Association guidelines for management of intracerebral haemorrhage therefore state that DNR orders should not be made within the first 48 hours, and that patients with DNR orders should continue to be given active treatment (25, 27).

It becomes increasingly clear that active management results in better outcomes. Ongoing studies will give us more answers. These include the TICH-2 study examining the effect of tranexamic acid as a haemostatic agent and the CLEAR III study of clot lysis for intraventricular haemorrhage.

3.3 Immediate access to advanced imaging and diagnostics

National stroke guidelines in the UK recommend that brain imaging should be performed within one hour of arrival under the following conditions: if there are indications for thrombolysis or early anticoagulation; if there is a known reversible bleeding risk (to exclude a haemorrhage); or if a non-vascular cause is suspected. These criteria are fulfilled in approximately 50% of acute strokes, with CT scanning recommended in the remainder as soon as possible within 24 hours (28). Immediate access to CT scanning for all patients presenting with acute stroke is practised in many units in Europe and the US. Early universal scanning has been established as a more effective and cost-effective diagnostic strategy than early scanning only for patients with specific indications (29). Further, more advanced imaging techniques, such as CT angiogram, CT perfusion, and magnetic resonance imaging, allow rapid and accurate diagnosis of the site of the occlusion and viability of the ischaemic penumbra, and therefore facilitate therapeutic decision making. This is supported by evidence from a meta-analysis of stroke-unit trials which showed that 24/7 availability of MRI scanning was associated with better outcomes (30).

3.4 Seven-day specialist stroke ward rounds

In the UK stroke services are covered by geriatricians; until recently services were provided on weekdays only with emergency cover for out-of-hours and weekends. This inevitably created capacity problems with infrequent discharges and consequently few acute stroke beds available during the weekend. Introduction of thrombolysis as a hyperacute treatment required 24/7 availability, and this is now considered standard for acute and hyperacute stroke units. In the third quarter of 2012, 40% of stroke patients admitted to English hospitals had a CT head scan within one hour, and 66% were admitted to the stroke unit within four hours of arrival at hospital (31). While the rationale for weekend ward rounds is assessment of new patients, follow-up of thrombolyzed patients, and facilitation of discharges, another important but often overlooked benefit is early diagnosis and treatment of complications in patients beyond the hyperacute phase. A retrospective cohort study of 96,621 patients with acute stroke admitted to UK hospitals over one year showed significantly higher mortality (OR 1.26, 95% CI: 1.16–1.37), more pneumonias, and fewer home discharges in patients admitted over the weekend (32). Increased mortality (OR 1.22, 95% CI: 1.00–1.25) for stroke patients admitted on weekends was also found in the Canadian stroke register in both mild and severe strokes, and even in transient ischaemic attacks (33). While in the UK series fewer weekend patients were scanned early and thrombolyzed, there was no difference in early scanning in the Canadian series. These numbers make a strong case for daily specialist ward rounds and 24/7 availability of key investigations.

3.5 Good nursing care

Most patients with severe stroke do not die of the neurological deficit itself, but of secondary complications such as dehydration, malnutrition, urinary tract infections, and, most importantly, pneumonia. The European Stroke Organization's recommendations for stroke units provide ample information on diagnostics and medical treatments, but nursing care is mentioned only in passing and with little detail (10). The evidence, however, suggests that nursing interventions may be considerably more important than medical treatments in determining mortality after stroke (34). Among seven care processes examined, treatment of all episodes of hypoxia was the most important intervention. A further retrospective study of the number of required processes of care delivered and complications demonstrated an inverse dose response relationship between the two. The single most important care process was early mobilization, which more than halved complications: significant effects were found on pneumonia, urinary tract infections, pressure sores, and constipation, but not on falls or thromboembolism (35). Data from the US Get with the Guidelines programme also suggest that dysphagia screening significantly reduces pneumonia (36). While these studies were all retrospective, randomized trials such as the AVERT phase III study of early mobilization are ongoing and will provide better evidence on the most effective interventions.

3.6 **Pneumonia prevention and management**

A meta-analysis including more than 10,000 stroke patients showed an incidence of 10% of stroke-associated pneumonia with a more than threefold increase of risk of death (37). Pneumonia is the most common cause of death after stroke: three times as many patients die of pneumonia than of stroke-related brain damage and the neurological deficit itself. The main cause of stroke-associated pneumonia is dysphagia and aspiration. There is strong evidence that screening for dysphagia reduces pneumonia (38). While there is still doubt that medical interventions such as prophylactic antibiotics can prevent infections (39), and large studies such as STRAWINSKI (40) are still ongoing there is increasing evidence that quality nursing care is key. This applies even very early on, in the emergency department, where mortality and pneumonia incidence is higher during nurse shift changes (41). Proactive management of dysphagia, early mobilization, and passive mobilization in bed are all associated with significant reductions in pneumonia.

3.7 **Prevention of venous thromboembolism**

Use of compressive stockings and prophylactic anticoagulation alone or in combination have been a key aspect of organized stroke care from its inception. The stockings were rapidly abandoned in 2009 after the CLOTS-1 study (42) demonstrated that they were ineffective. Prophylactic anticoagulation is still commonly used, although a recent meta-analysis has shown that prevention of pulmonary embolism is balanced by an increase in symptomatic intracerebral haemorrhage, with no overall long-term benefit (43). Furthermore, there is no evidence that long-term outcomes (death and disability) are better with the newer low-molecular heparins or heparinoids. The CLOTS-3 study demonstrated in 2013 that foot pumps effectively prevent venous thromboembolism. These pumps are also one of only three treatments (the others being stroke units and decompressive hemicraniectomy) which reduce mortality after stroke (44).

It remains to be seen whether these results will change clinical practice to the same extent as CLOTS-1, as many consider the devices cumbersome.

3.8 Avoidance of urinary catheters

Urinary tract infections are among the most common complications of stroke (45) and the majority are related to the insertion of urinary catheters. Catheterization is also associated with urosepsis (46) and an increase in mortality (47). Yet urinary catheters are still used regularly in acute stroke care, in spite of clear guidance to avoid catheterization wherever possible (28). Indications for catheterization include retention, assessment of fluid balance, prevention of decubitus ulcers, and patient dignity. Apart from the very rare stroke patient with coexistent uncontrolled heart and kidney failure requiring close monitoring of urine output, longer-term catheterization should not be necessary. There is no evidence that incontinence, properly managed with pads, causes skin breaks, as demonstrated in a large number of infants exposed to years of this method of containment. Uninfected urine is more sterile than saliva and has an acid pH which aids skin integrity. Urea, a key component of urine, softens both leather and skin. This is reflected in usage in the cosmetics industry, where, for example, urea is included in formulations of skin care products such as pH5 Eucerin. There is also no evidence that the presence of a catheter enhances dignity, especially as a pad may be hidden under clothing, whereas a catheter bag is usually visible to all. Patient views on this subject have not been studied. Urinary retention can be reversed by avoidance of anticholinergic medications, treatment of faecal impaction, and, in men, alpha one receptor antagonists, such as tamsolusin. Where this does not suffice, intermittent catheterization is less likely to cause infection. Unlike pneumonia, which is now attracting research interest, there are very few studies on the management of incontinence after stroke. The ICONS study is a start.

4 Future developments

While there has been a plethora of studies on acute stroke management and organization of stroke services, much still needs to be resolved. Stroke research is becoming part of standard clinical care, with 81% of UK stroke units taking part in one or more research studies (48) and with 7% of all stroke patients enrolled in trials (49). Finding faster and better ways to unblock occluded arteries and stopping bleeding in leaking arteries will continue to be at the forefront of research and development. There is, however, also an urgent need to improve the evidence base for nursing practice and rehabilitation. Such studies are often complex, with difficult-to-define interventions: it is easier to standardize a dose of a drug than a therapeutic session. However, the number and quality of studies in this field is growing. Examples include AVERT (early mobilization); Head-PoST (positioning in bed); and FAST INdIcATE (upper-limb therapy). Simple, widely applicable interventions, such as oxygen treatment (SO_2S study) and control of body temperature, are currently under investigation and could have wide-ranging effects. Finally, we will have to look beyond the acute and rehabilitation phase and address chronic problems and long-term consequences of stroke.

5 **Conclusion**

Unlike in the field of geriatric medicine, research has advanced rapidly in stroke medicine. This has led to major changes in treatment and service delivery, with ineffective treatments (compressive stockings) abandoned and effective interventions (thrombolysis and stroke unit care) implemented. It is becoming increasingly clear that rapid and accurate diagnosis of stroke and the identification of risk factors and complications are associated with better outcomes. While it remains unclear exactly what makes up the 'black box' of stroke-unit care, a willingness to find new solutions and subject these, and traditional standard practices, to scrutiny in clinical trials is likely to be important for the future.

Websites relevant to this chapter

The Internet Stroke Centre—resource for professionals

<http://www.strokecenter.org/professionals/>

The Internet Stroke Centre—patient resource

<http://www.strokecenter.org/patients/>

The European Stroke Organization website

<http://www.eso-stroke.org/>

The Karolinska Consensus Statements on Stroke Treatment

<http://www.strokeupdate.org/previous.aspx>

The Stroke Association (UK)

<http://www.stroke.org.uk/>

Stroke in Stoke—key documents and links

<http://www.stroke-in-stoke.info/>

Key guidelines, policy documents, and reviews

Stroke unit 'black box'

European Stroke Organization recommendations to establish a stroke unit and stroke center. (2013)

Revised and updated recommendations for the establishment of primary stroke centers: a summary statement from the Brain Attack Coalition. (2011)

British Association of Stroke Physicians stroke service standards. (2010)

Acute ischaemic stroke and transient ischaemic attack

Early management of patients with acute ischemic stroke: American Heart Association/American Stroke Association guidance. (January 2013)

Management of acute ischaemic stroke and TIA guidance from Royal College of Physicians. (October 2012)

Intracerebral haemorrhage

Management of spontaneous intracerebral hemorrhage: American Heart Association/American Stroke Association guidance. (January 2013)

References

1 **Stroke Unit Trialists.** Organised inpatient (stroke unit) care for stroke. Cochrane Database Syst Rev. 2007(4):CD000197.

2 **Langhorne P, Williams BO, Gilchrist W, Howie K.** Do stroke units save lives? Lancet. 1993. 342(8868):395–8.

3 **Stegmayr B, Asplund K, Hulter-Asberg K, Norrving B, Peltonen M, et al.** Riks-Stroke Collaboration. Stroke units in their natural habitat: can results of randomized trials be reproduced in routine clinical practice? Stroke. 1999;30(4):709–14.

4 **Seenan P, Long M, Langhorne P.** Stroke units in their natural habitat: systematic review of observational studies. Stroke. 2007;38(6):1886–92.

5 **Ko KF, Sheppard L.** The contribution of a comprehensive stroke unit to the outcome of Chinese stroke patients. Singapore Med J. 2006;47(3):208–12.

6 **Suwanwela NC, Eusattasak N, Phanthumchinda K, Piravej K, Locharoenkul C.** Combination of acute stroke unit and short-term stroke ward with early supported discharge decreases mortality and complications after acute ischemic stroke. J Med Assoc Thai. 2007;90(6):1089–96.

7 **Alberts MJ, Latchaw RE, Selman WR, Shephard T, Hadley MN, et al.** Recommendations for comprehensive stroke centers: a consensus statement from the Brain Attack Coalition. Stroke. 2005;36(7):1597–616.

8 **Alberts MJ, Hademenos G, Latchaw RE, et al.** Recommendations for the establishment of primary stroke centers. JAMA-J Am Med Assoc. 2000;283(23):3102–9.

9 **Alberts MJ, Latchaw RE, Jagoda A, Wechsler LR, Crocco T, et al.** Revised and updated recommendations for the establishment of primary stroke centers: a summary statement from the Brain Attack Coalition. Stroke. 2011;42(9):2651–6510.

10 **Ringelstein EB, Chamorro A, Kaste M, Langhorne P, Leys D, et al.** European Stroke Organisation recommendations to establish a stroke unit and stroke center. Stroke. 2013;44(3):828–40.

11 **Cassidy T, Roffe C, Keir S, Cloud G, Collas D, et al.** British Association of Stroke Physicians. Stroke service standards 2010. Accessed 28 May 2014. http://www.basp.ac.uk/Portals/2/2010 BASP Stroke Service Standards.pdf

12 **Price C, Emsley HC, Roffe C, Robinson T, James M.** Consultant workforce requirements 2011–5. British Association of Stroke Physicians 2011. Accessed 28 May 2014.

http://www.basp.ac.uk/Portals/2/BASP Meeting the Future Challenge of Stroke 2011-15.pdf

13 **Stroke Unit Trialists' Collaboration.** Organised inpatient (stroke unit) care for stroke. Cochrane Database Syst Rev. 2007(4):CD000197.

14 **National Institute of Neurological Disorders and Stroke rt-PA Stroke Study Group.** Tissue plasminogen activator for acute ischemic stroke. N Engl J Med. 1995; **333**(24):1581–8.

15 **Hacke W, Kaste M, Bluhmki E, Brozman M, Dávalos A, et al.** Thrombolysis with alteplase 3 to 4.5 hours after acute ischemic stroke. N Engl J Med. 2008;**359**(13): 1317–29.

16 **IST-3 Collaborative Group.** The benefits and harms of intravenous thrombolysis with recombinant tissue plasminogen activator within 6 h of acute ischaemic stroke (the third international stroke trial [IST-3]): a randomised controlled trial. Lancet. 2012;**379**(9834):2352–2363.

17 **Lally F, Grunwald IQ, Sanyal R, Natarajan I, Roffe C.** Mechanical thrombectomy in acute ischaemic stroke: a review of the literature, clinical effectiveness and future use. CNS Neurol Disord Drug Targets. 2013;**12**(2):170–90.

18 **Chimowitz MI.** Endovascular treatment for acute ischemic stroke—still unproven. N Engl J Med. 2013;**368**(10):952–5.

19 **Vahedi K, Hofmeijer J, Juettler E, Vicaut E, George B, et al.** Early decompressive surgery in malignant infarction of the middle cerebral artery: a pooled analysis of three randomised controlled trials. Lancet Neurol. 2007;**6**(3):215–22.

20 **Jüttler E, Unterberg A, Woitzik J, Bösel J, Amiri H, et al.** DESTINY II Investigators. Hemicraniectomy in older patients with extensive middle-cerebral-artery stroke. N Engl J Med. 2014;**370**(12):1091–100.

21 **Ronning OM, Guldvog B, Stavem K.** The benefit of an acute stroke unit in patients with intracranial haemorrhage: a controlled trial. J Neurol Neurosurg Psychiat. 2001;**70**(5):631–4.

22 **Feigin VL, Anderson N, Rinkel GJ, Algra A, van Gijn J, et al.** Corticosteroids for aneurysmal subarachnoid haemorrhage and primary intracerebral haemorrhage. Cochrane Database Syst Rev. 2005(3):CD004583.

23 **Mendelow AD, Gregson BA, Fernandes HM, Murray GD, Teasdale GM, et al.** Early surgery versus initial conservative treatment in patients with spontaneous supratentorial intracerebral haematomas in the International Surgical Trial in Intracerebral Haemorrhage (STICH): a randomised trial. Lancet. 2005;**365**(9457):387–97.

24 **Mendelow AD, Gregson BA, Rowan EN, Murray GD, Gholkar A, et al.** Early surgery versus initial conservative treatment in patients with spontaneous supratentorial lobar intracerebral haematomas (STICH II): a randomised trial. Lancet. 2013;**382**(9890): 397–408.

25 **Morgenstern LB, Hemphill JC III, Anderson C, Becker K, Broderick JP, et al.** Guidelines for the management of spontaneous intracerebral hemorrhage: a guideline for healthcare professionals from the American Heart Association/American Stroke Association. Stroke. 2010;**41**(9):2108–29.

26 **Anderson CS, Heeley E, Huang Y, Wang J, Stapf C, et al.** Rapid blood-pressure lowering in patients with acute intracerebral hemorrhage. N Engl J Med. 2013;**368**(25):2355–65.

27 Hemphill JC III, Newman J, Zhao S, Johnston SC. Hospital usage of early do-not-resuscitate orders and outcome after intracerebral hemorrhage. Stroke. 2004;**35**(5):1130–4.

28 Intercollegiate Stroke Working Party. National clinical guidelines for stroke. 4th ed. London: Royal College of Physicians; 2012.

29 Wardlaw JM, Seymour J, Cairns J, Keir S, Lewis S, et al. Immediate computed tomography scanning of acute stroke is cost-effective and improves quality of life. Stroke. 2004;**35**(11):2477–83. Epub 2004 Sep 30.

30 Candelise L, Gattinoni M, Bersano A, Micieli G, Sterzi R, et al. Stroke-unit care for acute stroke patients: an observational follow-up study. Lancet. 2007;**369**(9558): 299–305.

31 Intercollegiate Stroke Working Party. Stroke Improvement National Audit Programme (SINAP). Seventh Quarterly Public Report. Royal College of Physicians, London. Accessed 15 Aug 2013. http://www.rcplondon.ac.uk/sites/default/files/national_sinap_7th_quarterly_public_report_oct_-_dec_2012_admissions_0.pdf

32 Palmer WL, Bottle A, Davie C, Vincent CA, Aylin P. Dying for the weekend: a retrospective cohort study on the association between day of hospital presentation and the quality and safety of stroke care. Arch Neurol. 2012;**69**(10):1296–302.

33 Fang J, Saposnik G, Silver FL, Kapral MK. Association between weekend hospital presentation and stroke fatality. Neurology. 2010;**75**(18):1589–96.

34 Bravata DM, Wells CK, Lo AC, Nadeau SE, Melillo J, et al. Processes of care associated with acute stroke outcomes. Arch Intern Med. 2010. **170**(9):804–10.

35 Ingeman A, Andersen G, Hundborg HH, Svendsen ML, Johnsen SP. Processes of care and medical complications in patients with stroke. Stroke. 2011;**42**(1):167–72.

36 Masrur S, Smith EE, Saver JL, Reeves MJ, Bhatt DL, et al. Dysphagia screening and hospital-acquired pneumonia in patients with acute ischemic stroke: findings from Get with the Guidelines-stroke. J Stroke Cerebrovasc Dis. 2013;**22**(8):e301–9.

37 Westendorp W, Nederkoorn P, Vermeij J-D, Dijkgraaf M, van de Beek D. Post-stroke infection: A systematic review and meta-analysis. BMC Neurol. 2011;**11**(1):1–7.

38 Hinchey JA, Shephard T, Furie K, Smith D, Wang D, et al. Formal dysphagia screening protocols prevent pneumonia. Stroke. 2005;**36**(9):1972–6.

39 Meisel A, Meisel C, Harms H, Hartmann O, Ulm L. Predicting post-stroke infections and outcome with blood-based immune and stress markers. Cerebrovasc Dis. 2012;**33**(6):580–8.

40 Ulm L, Ohlraun S, Harms H, Hoffmann S, Klehmet J, et al. STRoke Adverse outcome is associated WIth NoSocomial Infections (STRAWINSKI): procalcitonin ultrasensitive-guided antibacterial therapy in severe ischaemic stroke patients—rationale and protocol for a randomized controlled trial. Int J Stroke. 2013;**8**(7):598–603.

41 Jones EM, Albright KC, Fossati-Bellani M, Siegler JE, Martin-Schild S. Emergency department shift change is associated with pneumonia in patients with acute ischemic stroke. Stroke. 2011;**42**(11):3226–30.

42 CLOTS (Clots in Legs Or sTockings after Stroke) Trials Collaboration. Effectiveness of thigh-length graduated compression stockings to reduce the risk of deep vein thrombosis after stroke (CLOTS trial 1): a multicentre, randomised controlled trial. Lancet. 2009;**373**(9679):1958–65.

43 **Geeganage CM, Sprigg N, Bath MW, Bath PM.** Balance of symptomatic pulmonary embolism and symptomatic intracerebral hemorrhage with low-dose anticoagulation in recent ischemic stroke: a systematic review and meta-analysis of randomized controlled trials. J Stroke Cerebrovasc Dis. 2013;**22**(7):1018–27.

44 **CLOTS (Clots in Legs Or sTockings after Stroke) Trials Collaboration.** Effectiveness of intermittent pneumatic compression in reduction of risk of deep vein thrombosis in patients who have had a stroke (CLOTS 3): a multicentre randomised controlled trial. Lancet. 2013;**382**(9891):516–21.

45 **Indredavik BF, Rohweder GF, Naalsund E, Lydersen S.** Medical complications in a comprehensive stroke unit and an early supported discharge service. Stroke. 2008;**39**(2):414–20.

46 **Warren JW.** Catheter-associated urinary tract infections. Infect Dis Clin North Am. 1997;**11**(3):609–22.

47 **Kwan J, Hand P.** Infection after acute stroke is associated with poor short-term outcome. Acta Neurol Scand. 2007;**115**(5):331–8.

48 **Intercollegiate Stroke Working Party.** National Sentinel Stroke Audit. Organisational Audit 2010. London: Royal College of Physicians. Accessed 28 May 2014. http://www. rcplondon.ac.uk/sites/default/files/public_organisational_report_2010.pdf

49 **Intercollegiate Stroke Working Party.** National Sentinel Stroke Clinical Audit 2010. Round 7. London: Royal College of Physicians; 2012. Accessed 28 May 2014. http:// www.rcplondon.ac.uk/sites/default/files/national-sentinel-stroke-audit-2010-public-report-and-appendices_0.pdf

Chapter 15

Involving older people in the design and conduct of clinical trials:
what is patient and public involvement?

Kate Wilde and Zena Jones

Key points

- There are strong policy drivers in the UK to involve patients not only as participants in research, but also as members of the research team.
- Patient and public involvement (PPI) can have significant benefits to the patient as well as to the research project.
- Many research funders require PPI explicitly described and evaluated in research proposals.
- Researchers need increased awareness of PPI, guidance, and a framework of how best to implement PPI within their research strategies.
- There is a risk of 'tokenistic' involvement of service users.
- There is the potential for a power struggle between the PPI representative with personal experience and the lead researcher with academic knowledge of the condition studied.
- There is a need to formally evaluate the impact of PPI on the effectiveness of research to bring new treatments to patients.

1 Introduction

The views of customers or service users, expressed by 'voting with their feet' (or wallets), clearly have an impact on the success of a business. However, where there is a monopoly, this mechanism of quality control is considerably weakened. The introduction of a national health service created such a monopoly and therefore risks losing contact with service users. The notion that patients could be regarded as consumers was promoted by the publication of the consultative paper 'Patients First' in 1979 (1). An attempt to rename patients as consumers has been unsuccessful in the health service, although social services introduced and kept the consumer-oriented term 'client' (2,3). The idea of active involvement of service users in the development and running of health services was introduced by the publication of 'Patient and Public Involvement in the New NHS' in 1999 (4). The benefits the Department of Health anticipated from involving patients are highlighted in this paper and summarized in Box 15.1. 'Patient experience' has since become an important driver in service development, design of governance standards, national service frameworks, and policy documents such as the 'Standards for Better Health' (2006) (5).

Since then this concept has become pervasive throughout the NHS, generating further publications and guidance (Box 15.2).

A consequence of the perceived success of patient involvement in the development and delivery of NHS is that policymakers question their

---

Box 15.1 Potential benefits of patient and public involvement in the health service

- **The patient perspective:** Patients are the experts in how they feel and what it is like to live with a condition.

- **Improving services:** By involving users and carers during planning and development, there is less risk of providing inappropriate services and more chance of services being provided in the way people want them.

- **Improving public understanding:** Greater openness, accountability, and involvement of the public should help to create a better understanding of complex NHS and health issues and strengthen public confidence in the NHS.

- **Improving health:** Involving people in influential decisions can improve their self-esteem, confidence, and overall well-being.

Text extract reproduced from NHS Executive. Patient and public involvement in the new NHS. Leeds: Department of Health; 1999. <http://webarchive.nationalarchives.gov.uk/+/www.dh.gov.uk/en/Publica tionsandstatistics/Lettersandcirculars/Healthservicecirculars/DH_ 4004176> (4) under the Open Government Licence v2.0.

> ## Box 15.2 Key publications relating to patient and public involvement in the health service
>
> ◆ Section 11 of the Health and Social Care Act (2001) indicates a statutory duty to consult and involve patients and the public (6).
>
> ◆ Patient and public involvement in health: The evidence for policy implementation (2004) (7).
>
> ◆ Our health, our care, our say: a new direction for community services (2006) (8).
>
> ◆ A stronger local voice: A framework for creating a stronger local voice in the development of health and social care services (2006) (9). These plans included the establishment of Local Involvement Networks (LINks) which replaced patient forums.
>
> ◆ An economic case for patient and public involvement (2012) (10).

attitude to patients in other aspects of the provision of health care. It is believed that active involvement of the public in the research process leads to more relevant, applicable research outcomes that result in improvements in practice in health and social care. When the Department of Health and the National Institute of Health Research set up the clinical research networks, involvement of service users, not only as subjects of research but as active members of the research team, became an integral part of the constitution of these organisations. Funders of research also recognized the importance of the patients' voice and required service-user input into research protocols, trial steering and management committees, and research dissemination (11,12). Some links to current guidance and views can be seen in the document and website sections at the end of the chapter. The 'Research Governance Framework for Health and Social Care' (13) requires the active involvement of service users and carers at every stage of research and promotes a move towards greater openness about research undertaken by organizations.

2 Defining and promoting patient and public involvement

Patient and public involvement (PPI) requires the active participation of service users in the development and management of the research project, rather than the participation as a subject of the research. While some patients may engage in research in several roles—subject and advisor, for example—only the advisory element is regarded as PPI. PPI can occur at several levels; these are:

1 Consultation—Patients and public are asked to comment on the design, the wording, and overall look and feel of research proposals, documents, and policy material. While much input may be sought, the role is mainly editorial: the critique of materials that have already been written on a topic that has been decided upon by professionals.

2 Collaboration—Patients and the public are involved in the design, strategic decisions, and the generation of a concept, and are partners and co-members of the research team.

3 Patient- and public-led research—Patients and members of the public generate and develop the research idea. They are the lead researchers and the rest of the research team support them to design a protocol and funding proposal, recruit patients, analyze data, etc.

Presently most PPI involves a combination of collaboration and consultation; although patient-led research is seen as the pinnacle of PPI, this remains relatively rare (14).

The organization INVOLVE was set up through a Department of Health initiative to ensure active public involvement in research and development in the NHS. Their remit is to:

- promote the empowerment of the public to become more involved in research
- develop alliances between the public, researchers, the Department of Health, and other research funders and sponsors in order to promote greater public involvement in research
- monitor public involvement in research
- encourage the evaluation of the effects of public involvement in research.

INVOLVE reports to the Department of Health on progress, and makes recommendations about the development of public involvement in research. Their policies are outlined on their website (<www.invo.org.uk>), which also provides guidance documents and evidence for the effectiveness of PPI.

There is therefore no doubt that the relevance of patient and public involvement in research is accepted by policymakers in the UK, but while the underlying rationale is convincing, it will be important to examine whether this has had any impact on the quality of research and the implementation of results. Scepticism exists among health care professionals, researchers, and members of the public.

3 **Role of older people in patient and public involvement in research**

There is a growing body of publications examining PPI in research relating to older people (15–25). In addition, the National Institute for Health Research clinical research networks collect case stories to illustrate benefits and issues (Boxes 15.3–15.5). The following themes emerge from this literature:

+ Involving older people in research benefits researchers.
+ This ensures the outcomes of the research are more applicable to the health care setting and patient group.
+ Older people may provide greater insight and qualitative data on issues.
+ Their involvement can benefit the quality of the research data.
+ Older people themselves benefit from being involved.
+ Provision of training and support to older people is essential.
+ Involvement of older people helps to challenge stereotypes and ageism, and promotes a positive image for older people.
+ Researchers need to be aware of and guard against tokenism.
+ PPI takes time and this needs to be planned for in a project.

These themes are explored further in the following sections.

4 **What are the benefits of PPI?**

This section discusses the benefits of PPI in relation to older people along with the potential and actual benefits to the research team, the quality of the research, and implementation of results into clinical practice.

4.1 **Benefits to older people who get involved**

Analysis of the evidence outlined in section 2 of this chapter suggests that PPI has a number of benefits for older people involved in research. These include the chance to meet new people, visit new places, and redevelop social skills. The

---

Box 15.3　My research journey

In this video a stroke survivor describes how getting involved in research has assisted with his rehabilitation and has opened up new opportunities for him, socially and intellectually. Video link: <http://www.youtube.com/watch?v=fWNNhieJ00g>

Box 15.4 The critical friend: some quotes from PPI groups

'Like the little boy in "The Emperor's Suit of Clothes" they will tell you when you are naked. Older people are particularly astonishing in this regard. I have seen a PPI member play along with the "nice old gentleman" image until something tries to slide past them. Suddenly you have the retired CEO of a multinational company in the room. Didn't see that coming!'

'We had a trial proposal come to us, needed PPI review urgently, last-minute, before the deadline for submission. We got a PPI panel together and reviewed it. They nodded politely when we told them their plan was flawed and that they would never recruit patients at the stage in the pathway they were aiming for. They submitted it anyway. It was rejected and they shared the feedback. Reviewers said the same as we did. Ignore us at your peril!'

'The research was involving restricting the use of a person's good arm in order to force them to mobilize their affected arm. I was nearly in tears when the researcher described this to me. Don't they know how frustrating that would feel?'

'You're recruiting patients at three months? I wasn't able to focus on my rehabilitation for at least a year.'

Box 15.5 Principles of PPI

- The roles of consumers are agreed between the researchers and consumers involved in the research.
- Researchers budget appropriately for the costs of consumer involvement in research.
- Researchers respect the differing skills, knowledge, and experience of consumers.
- Consumers are offered training and personal support to enable them to be involved in research.
- Researchers ensure that they have the necessary skills to involve consumers in the research process.
- Consumers are involved in decisions about how participants are both recruited and kept informed about the progress of the research.
- Consumer involvement is described in research reports.
- Research findings are available to consumers in formats and in language they can easily understand.

case study in Box 15.3 endorses this observation, noting particularly how much the patient's dysphasia improved after getting involved.

Davis and Nolan (15) noted that the older people made new friends during their research involvement, built confidence, developed new skills, and had greater visibility. Loss of confidence and role in society can lead to older people feeling they are becoming invisible. This was highlighted by the case study of a 65-year-old woman who reported, 'When you get older you suddenly become invisible. You can walk into a shop and people just don't see you or hear you. I never thought it would be like that, never thought I would disappear.'

More importantly, PPI brings many patients and carers into intimate contact with each other and with current trends in research. We should remember, especially in the case of older people, the intellectual stimulation they used to get from working life. Leamy and Clough (16) describe older people's need for engagement in educational opportunities. Blair and Minkler (17) highlight how involvement improved the knowledge and understanding of both researchers and the older people involved. Opportunities may arise for people to gain specific transferable skills or qualifications. Taylor (18) discussed the research training needs of older people and recommended user-friendly, non-accredited research training and specific support to enable research involvement, whereas Leamy and Clough (16) commented on older people's participation in formal research training.

It is worth highlighting a conflicting view here. Taylor (18) asked older people what they wanted and thought they needed to gain skills to become more involved in research; the older people talked about support and less formal training. However, Leamy and Clough (16) were looking at formal training for members of the public and what education was needed to transform a lay person into a functional researcher. This was based more on what a research team would need a person to bring with them in terms of knowledge and skills. Both papers do, however, acknowledge the broad view that training and support is required for lay people to make a meaningful contribution as researchers. In terms of benefit to the older lay person, these skills and possibly qualifications may help them get more out of their involvement experience and enhance their credibility so that they are asked to be involved again in other projects.

Involvement may directly benefit the individual's condition, as described earlier in relation to dysphasia and also by Tanner (19) in work done with older people with dementia. In that study, older people with dementia were recruited as co-researchers and interviewers, collecting data from older research subjects with dementia. The co-researchers reported that their involvement gave them a sense of purpose and value, countering the feelings of powerlessness usually associated with dementia. Tetley et al. (20) describe how getting involved in research led to wider involvement opportunities for older people in their local communities and helped them make wider links and increase their sphere of influence. An added benefit was that other professionals approached the now experienced lay people to get involved with other projects, including service planning and community improvement projects.

Philanthropic reasons are another key motivator for PPI; some people just want to help others, as described by Leamy and Clough (16). These themes are not mutually exclusive and people may have a number of complex motivations to get involved in research.

4.2 **Benefits to researchers**

Expert patients, their families, and carers can provide valuable insight into the experience of living with a condition. The moral and ethical right of stakeholders to be actively involved in changes and developments that affect them—'nothing about us without us' (21)—is now broadly accepted. Many funding bodies now require grant proposals to explicitly describe the extent of PPI in the project development; PPI may thereby influence funding decisions. For example, the bodies responsible for funding research in the area of health technology assessment, as well as in the area of efficacy and mechanism evaluation, include patients and the public on their boards. The remit of these members includes critiquing the PPI in project proposals. Thus, promoters of PPI should be pushing at an open door. Despite inducements such as these, PPI remains limited and attitudes vary, as outlined by Thompson et al. (22). This is explored further in section 5 of this chapter.

Older people, in particular, may be in a position to make major contributions to research as they have a lifetime of knowledge and experience to share. Many are retired and are willing to give time to work with research teams, often for little or no financial compensation. There are also less obvious factors. Dewar (23) observed that one of the greatest impacts was that older people relate well to one another. This enabled recruitment of hard to reach groups, and inclusion of more in-depth interview material as subjects seemed to be more open in interviews with their peers. Additionally, information was disseminated more effectively back to older people by older people. Miller et al. (24) stated that involving older people in the early stages of research helped the researchers be clearer about their aims and shaped the development of the interview schedule. Davis and Nolan (15) noted that older people were able to focus the researchers on issues that are important to them. Finally, working closely with older people challenged myths and stereotypes about ageing.

4.3 **Benefits to research quality**

Some of the benefits to research quality are difficult to distinguish from researcher benefits, but there are some subtleties worth exploring. Ross et al. (25) noted that their advisory group of older people helped with developing interview schedules and also with validating methodology through independent observation of focus groups. The experiences people bring to the project can provide unexpected sources of expertise. Older people may have 'seen it all before' and spot obvious pitfalls in planning and execution of a project that a less experienced research team may not have anticipated. What may seem a practical and acceptable request to patients in a protocol may prove too difficult, painful, or impractical for the patient. Examples of this type of input are given in Box 15.4. Boote et al. (26) reported how PPI prevented a poor idea going forward. Although health professionals approved the idea, the PPI panel did not think it worth pursuing, it was therefore abandoned, ensuring that public money was not wasted. The authors of the paper felt this was as an important benefit of PPI. Another success story was recounted by Staniszewska et al. (27) who stated, 'Through careful collaboration a research bid was produced which was rooted in users' experiences, while addressing key research questions.' Anecdotally, a PPI committee member is said to have stated: 'It makes scientific sense to ensure that theories and assumptions ring true with users' experiences and expectations. Otherwise, whom are we doing this for?'

5 **Drawbacks, cautions, and future work**

Many commentaries and studies allude to difficulties with involving older people in research. Ross et al. (25) describe slippage of timescales and agendas as a result of PPI, but conceded that this may not be such a bad thing if the outcomes are better. Dewar (23) discussed the need to have a clear purpose for PPI, to know what involvement means, and to be critical about the importance of involving users in research. Dewar also stressed the need to manage expectations of the users. The difference between research and service development is not always obvious to members of the public—until they see that the research they are involved in will not change the way services are delivered overnight. Researchers often cite the need for a framework, structure, or guideline. Other potential dangers with PPI have been highlighted in the literature. These include poor disability access, inadequate provision for carers, and lack of individual support and training (15–25). Staniszewska et al. (27) identified lack of financial support for users as a barrier to involvement. One also has to be careful of individuals who want to use the research forum as a platform to advance their specific cause or complaint. This needs careful management with group work, as it is not always obvious at the outset and it is important to ensure the research agenda stays on topic. Associated with this is the need to ensure that quieter members have their views heard. The use of skilled facilitators is essential in these circumstances. A seasoned facilitator will strike a balance in allowing some time for personal opinions before getting down to the purpose of the meeting.

Some research teams carefully recruit PPI members, issuing role descriptions and conducting interviews. The NIHR Stroke Research Network has adopted this practice for lay members of their clinical steering groups (view PPI strategy on their website <www.crn.nihr.ac.uk/stroke>). There may be issues over representation. Some groups will try hard to get the right demographic mix of ethnicity, age, social grouping, etc. Shea et al. (28) discussed the merits and drawbacks of using virtual PPI (discussion over email and other electronic media) as a means to get wider demographic and skill representation.

While much has been done politically to endorse PPI, it may not be getting through to researchers. Should more be done to promote PPI and make it easier to implement? The work of INVOLVE is on-message but are researchers aware of it? Perhaps it should be more explicitly incorporated into researcher training. Anecdotally, discussions with researchers new to PPI show that they are often at a loss to know where to begin. They are unsure how they can involve people, at what stage, and how much time and money will be required. Research managers and NHS professionals can be equally unsure or unconvinced. There can also be a power struggle: professional researchers may be unwilling to relinquish the belief that their years of training and academic pursuit make their ideas more valuable than those of a service user. A very senior researcher was quoted as saying, 'I don't believe any member of the public could come up with an idea for research [into a specific condition] that my senior research colleagues and I haven't already thought of.' An unwillingness to confront some of these tensions head-on can lead to tokenistic involvement, box ticking, and ultimately low-impact, low-benefit PPI for all involved.

Many academics would like a manual that tells them all they need to know about PPI. Because such guidance already exists (29,30) (see also Box 15.5 and <www.invo.org.uk>), there may be a need to raise awareness. However, there is no absolute formula; each project needs a different approach and each set of individuals is unique. There is no substitute for a well thought out, project specific PPI strategy that is flexible enough to adapt to the changing needs of all the professional and non-professional researchers.

The dearth of research activity on the impact of PPI, particularly involving older people, is both a source of concern and of opportunity. This is clearly an area which needs further exploration and expansion. The public and the Department of Health may both want more projects to explicitly involve older people at every stage but, more than ever, as budgets get squeezed, any activity which absorbs resources must demonstrate tangible impact and benefit. Evidence is available to support PPI in research for older people but it requires further strengthening and publicity. Box 15.6 describes two ongoing pre-publication projects which will hopefully add to the evidence base in time. At the time of writing, the authors were cheered to see a publication from Ennis and Wykes (31) with the incisive title 'Impact of Patient Involvement in Mental Health Research: Longitudinal Study.' The paper concludes that mental health studies with associated PPI were significantly more successful at achieving recruitment targets than those without PPI. They recommend further research to explore this finding.

6 **Conclusion**

The evidence appears to show that involving older people in research benefits the researchers, the older people who choose to get involved, and the research quality. However, the evidence is based on few studies and case reports, and

---

Box 15.6 **Up and coming work: two projects pre-publication**

- SAFER 2 trial (Support and Assessment for Falls Emergency Referrals): Bridie Evans, Swansea University, HTA-funded project
  - The trial is a cluster randomized control involving ambulance services which are randomized to provide usual care or paramedic assessment and referral to a community falls-prevention service. Older people who have experienced falls are involved in overseeing the trial both centrally and as a local resource to the sites and in supporting the site research teams by discussing issues facing older people.
- The PEOPPLE project (Putting Evidence for Older People into Practice in Living Environments): Karen Burnell, University of Portsmouth, HEIF-funded project
  - The project aims to identify unmet needs of older people in Portsmouth. The project consults with older people's groups to identify unmet needs and research priorities, and to develop community-based projects. Older people have been involved at every stage; the project has so far involved 96 members of the public, giving 656 hours of their time.

publication bias cannot be excluded. The evidence base needs to be strengthened by a systematic review of tangible impacts.

Websites relevant to this chapter

TwoCan Associates. An evaluation of the COMPASS masterclass in consumer involvement in research. (2011)

<http://www.ncri.org.uk/publications/collaborate-and-succeed-an-evaluation-of-the-compass-masterclass-in-consumer-involvement-in-research>

NIHR Mental Health Research Network. Good practice guidance for involving carers, family members and close friends of service users in research. (2006)

http://www.crn.nihr.ac.uk/mentalhealth/

NIHR Diabetes Research Network. Patient and public involvement working group annual report. (2012–13)

http://www.drn.nihr.ac.uk/ppi/doc/ppiwg-annual-rep-2012-13.pdf

INVOLVE

Guidance, a repository of relevant research, and a list of ongoing projects

<www.invo.org.uk>

Key guidelines, policy documents, and reviews

Introduction of the concept of PPI to the NHS: Department of Health. Patient and public involvement in the new NHS. (4)

Discussion paper and analysis: Medical Research Council. Involving patients and the public can benefit clinical research. (11)

Guidance: Building on success: opportunities to progress patient and public involvement in research prioritization and commissioning. (12)

Guidance: Principles and indicators of successful consumer involvement in NHS research: results of a Delphi study and subgroup analysis. (29)

References

1 **Department of Health and Social Security (DHSS).** Patients first: consultative paper on the structure and management of the National Health Service in England and Wales. London: HMSO; 1979. Accessed 30 Sep 2013. Referenced in http://www.ncbi.nlm.nih.gov/pmc/articles/PMC1597459/

2 **The National Health Service and Community Care Act.** London: HMSO; 1990. Accessed 30 Sep 2013. http://www.legislation.gov.uk/ukpga/1990/19/contents

3 **Webster C.** The National Health Service: a political history. Oxford: Oxford University Press; 2002. p. 140–207.

4 **NHS Executive.** Patient and public involvement in the new NHS. Leeds: Department of Health; 1999. Accessed 30 Sep 2013. http://webarchive.nationalarchives.gov.uk/+/www.

dh.gov.uk/en/Publicationsandstatistics/Lettersandcirculars/Healthservicecirculars/
DH_4004176

5 **Department of Health**. Standards for better health. London: HMSO; 2006. Updated version. Gateway 6405. Accessed 29 Sep 2013. http://webarchive.nationalarchives.gov.uk/+/
dh.gov.uk/en/publicationsandstatistics/publications/publicationspolicyandguidance/
dh_4086665

6 **Health and Social Care Act**. London: HMSO; 2001. Accessed 29 Sep 2013.http://www.
legislation.gov.uk/ukpga/2001/15/contents

7 **Farrell C**. Patient and public involvement in health: the evidence for policy implementation. London: Department of Health; 2004. Gateway2880. Accessed 29 Sep 2013. http://
webarchive.nationalarchives.gov.uk/+/dh.gov.uk/en/publicationsandstatistics/
publications/publicationspolicyandguidance/dh_4082332

8 **Department of Health: Our health, our care, our say: a new direction for community
services**. London: HMSO; 2006.

9 **Department of Health**. A stronger local voice: a framework for creating a stronger local
voice in the development of health and social care services. London: HMSO; 2006. Gateway 6759. Accessed 29 Sep 2013. http://webarchive.nationalarchives.gov.uk/
20130107105354/http://www.dh.gov.uk/prod_consum_dh/groups/dh_digitalassets/
@dh/@en/documents/digitalasset/dh_4137041.pdf

10 **Frontline and InHealth Associates**. Briefing note: an economic case for patient and
public involvement in commissioning. London: Department of Health; 2012

11 **Vale C, Thompson L, Murphy C, Forcat S, Hanley B**. Involvement of consumers in
studies run by the MRC Clinical Trials Unit: results of a survey. Trials. 2012(13):9.

12 **Cowan K**. Building on success—the report of an event organized by the Association of
Medical Research Charities, INVOLVE, and the James Lind Alliance. 2010. Accessed
29 Sep 2013. http://www.lindalliance.org/pdfs/JLA%20Internal%20Reports/Building_
on_Success_Final_23_Sept_10.pdf

13 **Department of Health**. Research governance framework for health and social care.
2nd ed. London: HMSO; 2005. Accessed 20 Sep 2013. https://www.gov.uk/government/
uploads/system/uploads/attachment_data/file/139565/dh_4122427.pdf

14 **Department of Health**. Let me in—I'm a researcher! London: HMSO; 2006. Ref.
273293. http://webarchive.nationalarchives.gov.uk/20130107105354/http:/www.dh.gov.
uk/en/Publicationsandstatistics/Publications/PublicationsPolicyAndGuidance/
DH_4132916

15 **Davis S, Nolan M**. Nurturing research partnerships with older people and their carers:
learning from experience. Qual Ageing-Policy Pract Res. 2003;**4**(4):2–5.

16 **Leamy M, Clough R**. How older people became researchers: training, guidance and
practice in action. York: Joseph Rowntree Foundation; 2006.

17 **Blair T, Minkler M**. Participatory action research with older adults: key principles in
practice. Gerontologist. 2009;**49**(5):652–62.

18 **Taylor S**. A new approach to empowering older people's forums: identifying barriers to
encourage participation. Practice. 2006;**18**(2):117–28.

19 **Tanner D**. Co-research with older people with dementia: experience and reflections:
J Ment Health. 2012;**21**(3):296–306.

20 **Tetley J, Haynes L, Hawthorne M, Odeyemi J, Skinner J, Smith J, Wilson D**. Older
people and research partnerships. Qual Ageing-Policy Pract Res. 2003;**4**(4):18–23.

21 **Department of Health**. Nothing about us without us. London: HMSO; 2001. Ref. 23588. http://webarchive.nationalarchives.gov.uk/+/www.dh.gov.uk/en/Publication sandstatistics/Publications/PublicationsPolicyAndGuidance/DH_4006200

22 **Thompson J, Barber R, Ward P, Boote J, Cooper C, Armitage C, Jones G**. Health researchers' attitudes towards public involvement in health research. Health Expectations. 2009;**12**(2):209–20.

23 **Dewar B**. Beyond tokenistic involvement and older people in research—a framework for future development and understanding. J Clin Nurs. 2005;**14**(3a):48–53.

24 **Miller E, Morrison J, Cook A**. Brief encounter: collaborative research between academic researchers and older researchers. Generations Rev. 2006;**16**(3/4):39–41.

25 **Ross F, Donovan S, Brearley S, Victor C, Cottee M, Crowther P, Clark E**. Involving older people in research: methodological issues. Health Social Care Community. 2005;**13**(3):268–75.

26 **Boote J, Dagleish M, Freeman J, Jones Z, Miles M, Rodgers H**. 'But is it a question worth asking?' A reflective case study describing how public involvement can lead to researchers' ideas being abandoned. Health Expectations. 2012 Jun;**17**(3):440–51. doi: 10.111/j.1369-7625.2012.00771.x

27 **Staniszewska S, Jones N, Newburn M, Marshall S**. User involvement in the development of a research bid: barriers, enablers and impacts. Health Expectations. 2007;**10**:173–83.

28 **Shea B, Santesso N, Qualman A, Heilberg T, Leong A, Judd M, Robinson V, Wells G, Tugwell P, and the Cochrane Musculoskeletal Consumer Group**. Consumer-driven health care: building partnerships in research. Health Expectations. 2005;**8**:352–9.

29 **Telford R, Boote J, Cooper C**. Principles and indicators of successful consumer involvement in NHS research: results of a Delphi study and subgroup analysis. In: Boote J, Barber R, Cooper C, eds. Health Policy. 2006 Feb;**75**(3):280–97.

30 **Oliver S, Rees R, Clarke-Jones L, Milne R, Oakley A, Gabbay J, Stein K, Buchanan P, Gyte G**. A multidimensional conceptual framework for analysing public involvement in health services research: Health Expectations. 2008;**11**(1):72–84.

31 **Ennis L, Wykes T**. Impact of patient involvement in mental health research: longitudinal study: Brit J Psychiat. 2013;**203**:381–6. doi: 10.1192/bjp.bp.112.119818

Chapter 16

Under-representation of older people in clinical trials

Gary H. Mills

Key points

- Older people, often with high levels of co-morbidity and polypharmacy, are increasing in number as the population ages.
- Study populations in clinical trials have often not mirrored the population that will consume the drugs or treatments being investigated.
- Regulators, ethics committees, and funding bodies must recognize the need for inclusion of older people and the complexities this imposes on investigators.
- Across all aspects of medicine, funding for research into how best to safely include older people in clinical trials is vital.
- Researchers should not be disadvantaged by designing studies to meet the needs of the age range of patients expected to receive the treatment being investigated; this should include provision for older people.

---

1 Introduction

Older patients consume a large proportion of all medications. In the USA, 88% of those aged 60 used at least one prescription drug, compared to 48% in the 20–59 age bracket. Of those aged 60 and over, 37% used five or more drugs, compared to 8% in the 20–59 age range (1).

As described in Chapter 1, the proportion of older people in the population is rising throughout the developed world. It is therefore imperative from a practical perspective as well as for humanitarian reasons that older people are kept fit and independent for as long as possible.

Part of this process is the provision of suitably developed medication and treatment. Despite this, older people have often been excluded from clinical trials (2), even though in many situations the drugs being tested are used by a population whose age range is higher than the trial population (3). It is vital that drugs are trialed on a population that is similar in age and co-morbidity during the study phase, rather than relying on later reports to determine if complications are reported. This is because drug metabolism is different in older people compared to the younger population. Furthermore, older people are more likely to be taking multiple medications thereby increasing the risk of adverse drug reactions (see Chapter 5).

Randomized controlled studies are the gold standard test of a treatment, but the difficulties in matching populations can cause real difficulty in recruitment. The result is that there is a tendency to look at the simplest possible group, which frequently does not include older people, who are more likely to have co-morbidities. Selecting the best control therapy may also be difficult, as may the selection of primary and secondary outcomes that are most suited to all age groups. For example, in younger surgical cases survival is the key outcome, but in older people the chances of the quality of life being affected adversely is usually much greater. Loss of independence, especially if this involves cognitive problems, would be something that older people might fear most and might justifiably be regarded as the primary outcome. Information on quality-of-life outcomes that might be more commonly affected in older people are vital to allow them to make informed decisions, and vital as well for the doctors trying to select the best forms of treatment. Studies need to be designed and powered with these objectives in mind.

Medical specialists in areas as diverse as neurology and critical care have emphasized the need to include older people in clinical trials and have also stressed that many diseases are more common in older people. They have called upon funders, governments, and ethics committees to examine this problem (4). A study of critical care trials looked at exclusion based on age, gender, and race in 17,000 patients screened for inclusion in a study of acute lung injury. Age over 75 was related to exclusion, some of which could be explained by a high level of co-morbidity. This is important because the average age of the critical care population is increasing, as is the age range for major surgical interventions (5). Older people and women have been under-represented in randomized controlled trials of acute coronary syndromes in the past and this continues to be the case (6). This is particularly important because 60% of deaths related to myocardial infarction occur in patients aged 75 or older (7), and post–myocardial infarction morbidity, including heart failure, are more frequent (8). In fact, one type of heart failure—heart failure with preserved ejection fraction—is a disorder that is largely confined to the over-60s, with a mean age of 75 years (9). In a UK study of incidence of heart failure, the rate increased with age (10), reaching 11.6 new cases per 1,000 in those aged 85 and older. Approximately 80% of all heart failure cases occur in individuals aged 65 or older (11). Despite this, only 15% of heart failure studies have included patients over 80 years of age (12).

There is evidence from surveys of medical and related staff that the absence of relevant outcome data makes prescribing and treating older people difficult and impacts on equity of care (13). This is regarded as a problem across much of Europe (14). In a study of more than 500 clinicians in nine European countries, 87% of respondents concluded that exclusion on the grounds of age alone was unjustified and 79% felt this caused difficulties for prescribers. Respondents from most countries felt that changes to regulation were needed to reform current practice (14).

2 **The evidence for under-representation**

Evidence from published studies has shown that trial populations have not matched the age range of the clinical population (<http://www.predicteu.org/Reports/PREDICT_WP1_Report.pdf>). In a meeting of an expert committee of the European Medicines Agency, it was stated that in this context, 'The drugs we are using in older people have not been properly evaluated' (15). A consequence of age not matching the actual treatment group is that gender also will not be appropriate. Women survive into old age more commonly than men and so failure to recruit in these age groups will also disproportionately impact women. The PREDICT group investigated this by examining currently ongoing studies in the area of heart failure therapy as a key disease process for older people (16). Access to the European Medicine Database of ongoing studies was very difficult at the time; therefore data from ongoing clinical trials of heart failure were extracted from the World Health Organization Clinical Trials Registry Platform (<http://www.who.int/ictrp/publications/en/>). The key outcome measure was the proportion of trials excluding patients by an arbitrary upper age limit or by other exclusion criteria that indirectly limited recruitment of older individuals. Exclusion criteria were categorized as justified or poorly justified. Of 251 trials investigating treatments for heart failure, 64 (25.5%) excluded patients by an arbitrary upper age limit not related to other factors. Exclusion of older people was significantly ($p = 0.007$) more common in trials conducted in the European Union (31 of 96, 32.3%) than in the United States (17 of 105, 16.2%). Overall, 109 trials (43.4%) on heart failure had one or more poorly justified exclusion criteria that could limit the inclusion of older individuals due to the association of these factors with age.

Exclusion of older people in ongoing trials was independently examined in 206 studies of treatment for Parkinson's disease. It was concluded that exclusion on the basis of upper age limit was common, especially in smaller studies, with 49% of studies having a mean upper age limit of 79 years (17).

3 Older people and clinical trials—barriers and promoters

3.1 Barriers

There are many reasons why older people may be excluded from clinical trials (Box 16.1). Exclusion of the elderly may be solely based on arbitrary age limits (18,19). Sometimes this is to satisfy a perceived or real requirement of ethics committees. This appears to be more common in interventional studies and, while possibly decreasing, particularly in the USA, it continues to be a major problem in Europe (20). There is evidence that ethics committees may be inconsistent. This is especially so when the area they are considering involves complex regulatory regimes such as the Mental Capacity Act, which deals with adults in England and Wales who lack capacity to give informed consent. Complexity may lead to exclusion of people who lack capacity, as investigators quickly learn which areas of research lead to confusion and delays in what is already a lengthy permission process (21).

Box 16.1 Barriers to research in older people

+ arbitrary age limits
+ inappropriate exclusion criteria that disproportionately affect older people
+ lack of resources to cope with cognitive deficits
+ restrictions on co-morbid conditions
+ restrictions on polypharmacy
+ complex regulation, not designed with research in mind
+ logistical issues, such as loss of income, timing, and transport
+ lack of provision for carers
+ under-resourcing to provide for the extra time needed to recruit and gather data from older people
+ lack of appreciation of extra needs by funding bodies
+ physician resistance to study protocol
+ communication barriers between community and hospital care
+ lack of recognition for clinicians involved.

In the UK it is often regarded as acceptable for a close family member to make a decision for the patient and proceed on that basis. This is helpful, but does mean that a suitable person may not be available and/or needs to be found in a timescale that fits in with the project's requirements. An independent mental capacity advocate (IMCA) might be appointed for patients who lack capacity and do not have someone who can act as a consultee. Unfortunately, the IMCA role is not designed with research facilitation as a primary aim. A guidance document on such appointments was issued in 2008 (22). The IMCA could be a doctor independent of the research team. Although this may be the preferred route in emergency situations, it is not always easy to show that a nominated consultee is totally independent. The IMCA does not affect research that is a clinical trial as laid out in the *Medicines for Human Use Regulations 2004*, which include similar principles for the involvement of a 'legal representative'.

Canadian studies of oncology patients involved in clinical trials found that age was an important barrier to recruitment, even though some older people may be easier to recruit because they lack the time pressures of those who are employed and are more prepared to attend follow-up visits. Physicians' perceptions, protocol eligibility criteria with restrictions on co-morbid conditions, and functional status to optimize treatment tolerability are the most important reasons resulting in the exclusion of older patients. Other barriers include the lack of social support and the need for extra time and resources to enrol these patients (23).

In the UK, the research approval process is a major hurdle, and many believe that the simplest route to data is the best. Co-morbidity and polypharmacy complicate studies, increasing the numbers needed to recruit to an adequately powered study. The need to cope with transport and to facilitate communication in patients who may have impaired hearing or sight may increase the cost, time, and the skills needed to conduct a study (24). There is also a need to protect vulnerable subjects from adverse events in a study of a treatment that has unpredicted consequences. Therefore, some would argue that a simple initial study followed by a later study covering the needs of the elderly is the safest compromise. Unfortunately this depends on a further study actually being completed, which is difficult to guarantee without some form of legal compulsion.

In his systematic review for PREDICT (3), Andrew Beswick identified 19 studies reporting promoters and barriers to participation of older people in clinical trials extending back 20 years. These included the lack of an obligation for pharmaceutical companies to promote randomized controlled trials in older people and even lack of personal recognition for the physician involved.

3.1.1 Physician endorsement

Physicians' perceptions of the implications of the trial for the patient are important (25,26). Physicians may not wish their patients to participate because the trial process requires extra time and resources or related practical difficulties. Alternatively, trials may have implications for loss of professional autonomy, impact on the patient-physician relationship, or present consent difficulties (24,27). In three surveys of patients with cancer, the endorsement of an oncologist was reported to be a factor in trial participation (28). Physicians might advise against participation if they felt their patients would show poor compliance (29) or if they thought a therapy was not the right one.

In some systems, insurance issues—either with regard to the study or health care—may present difficulties (27,30). Such practical barriers include insurance companies' needing to agree, on an case-by-case basis, to the protocol for a study taking place in a private hospital. The idea is that the companies would want to weigh the risks of any extra provision they may have to cover as a result of the trial. In the USA, there was a change in 2000 in the Department of Health and Human Services medicare reimbursement policy, which allowed payment of routine care costs of older patients in clinical trials.

3.1.2 Transport and logistical barriers

Obstacles may be presented by financial or employment implications, such as transport costs, loss of work time, and inconvenience for a carer. Sometimes the patients themselves play a carer's role, which could be compromised by a study.

3.1.3 Treatment risks

Patients may be unwilling to compromise their current health care (31,32) or fear new adverse effects (33). They may fear the trial treatment or be unable to come to terms with the idea that they are being experimented on or being randomly assigned to one or another type of therapy, rather than receiving the 'best' (33). This may be even more difficult when the intervention is of an emergency nature. In a study of women's experiences when participating in a randomized controlled trial in a critical situation, there was evidence that the stress of the situation made it difficult to absorb information, which in turn influenced the decision to proceed (34). This highlights the need to ensure that documentation is easy to understand and retain as well as the need for skilled explanation when the study is being conducted in a critical situation. Fear of a placebo is a major concern for many (33) who might otherwise agree to take part in a comparison of the current versus a new treatment.

3.1.4 Lack of knowledge of the disease process

Patients may misunderstand study information (31). Advice from family members and other lay opinions—which may or may not be accurate—could influence the willingness of people to participate in clinical trials. Some patients may be unaware of the ill health targeted in the clinical trial.

3.1.5 Lack of compulsion in study design

As mentioned earlier, there is no requirement that studies, whether designed by pharmaceutical companies or not, use populations that match the disease population. This creates another obstacle to inclusion of older people in trial design (35).

3.2 **Promoters**

Patients take part in studies for a number of reasons, including perceived health benefits for themselves, altruism, extra health care, and follow-up (Box 16.2) (36,37). Patients with a family history of disease may be more likely to take part.

Effective interventions found to increase recruitment include the following: culture-specific strategies in ethnic groups, open-trial designs, telephone reminders, and monetary incentives. Personalized letters were identified as a strategy for further investigation. Interventions found to be ineffective in increasing participation included use of staff other than clinicians, research staff site visits, advance postcards or telephone calls by a nurse, patient-preference trial designs, and payment to health care professionals (38).

Using simple and clear language in written documents helps recruitment. Because the sections are long, the current standard information sheet layout

---

Box 16.2 Promoters of research in older people

- altruism
- perceived benefits for the volunteer
- open-trial designs
- monetary reward for patients and volunteers
- logistic support such as help with transport or refunding of expenses
- home visits
- telephone reminders
- culture-specific strategies in ethnic groups.

used in England may not be the best for this purpose for patients less able to concentrate on new information. The documentation of a study should be critically examined to determine how patients interpret the information and choices presented to them (39). This should be done early so that, if necessary, modifications can be made. It is also important to train staff so they can explain the study to participants, including to those who may have limitations in seeing, hearing, or mental capacity.

Increasing the rate of recruitment of older people in clinical trials has important implications for research, not least of which is the reduction of selection bias. A study showed that in 14 consecutive published trials, for every three older patients screened, only one was retained (2).

3.2.1 Practical and logistical promoters

Telephone contact, in addition to sending a questionnaire through the post, increased rates by 10% (40). Poor transport is a barrier for patients and may affect clinicians' decisions on inclusion (41). Adequate provision of ramps, lifts, wheelchair access, and appropriate toilet facilities for people with mobility impairments need to be readily available, together with reimbursement of costs (37). Other forms of practical assistance should be explored, such as visits to the patient's home.

3.2.2 Involvement of medical and related staff

The study needs to be perceived as having a reasonable chance of benefitting patients (42), otherwise clinicians will not actively support it.

Good practice, good communication with clinical staff, good publicity (including posters) and well-planned breaks for patients are vital. It is also important to plan appointments around carers' needs. Good access and a pleasant research environment for patients is needed so that they (and carers) will be happy to return. Posters and leaflets in public and patient areas will also help patients and their families realize that research is normal practice (2). Involvement of general practice with community studies is vital to boost recruitment.

3.2.3 Communication within the health system

In many health care systems there is a division between the hospital and care in the community. Much of this is due to poor communication and a lack of continuity. This impacts on research, particularly in the areas of longer-term outcomes and research follow-up. Many hospital-based studies lack general practice involvement. This is partly because of the difficulty in reliably communicating the needs of a study from relatively small groups of hospital clinicians to the wider group of general practitioners in the locality, or even more widely for patients who are receiving tertiary treatment.

One way around these difficulties is primary care research networks, which enable GPs to screen and follow up patients for hospital-based or other studies. This requires careful planning and the inclusion of a research lead from general practice at the planning and grant application stage. The incorporation of research as a core activity of the health system might facilitate changes that would make the needs of research projects a routine consideration for all doctors. However, accommodating this with the authorities who are responsible for purchasing the health care may be complex and may change over time. Similarly, studies based in the community are often ignored once a patient is hospitalized. Timely follow-up in both directions would facilitate data gathering, but there is a great divide at present.

4 The EU Charter

The European Charter for Older People in Clinical Trials was aimed to publicize the exclusion of older people from clinical research and to influence research-related bodies such as research ethics committees and clinical trial organizers and funders (Box **16.3**). In 2010 the PREDICT group presented the initial version of the charter to a wide audience at British Medical Association (BMA) House in London. After further development it was presented to a meeting on the care of older people at the European Parliament in Brussels in 2011 (43) and launched, initially in 13 languages together with a lay version, the same year. The purpose of the charter was to encourage the adoption of rights for older people in clinical trials. The key points were the following: older people have the right to access evidence-based treatments; the inclusion of older people in clinical trials prevents a form of discrimination; clinical trials should

---

Box 16.3 Features of the European Charter for Older People in Clinical Trials (from the PREDICT group)

- Older people have the right to access evidence-based medicine.
- Inclusion of older people in clinical trials should be encouraged; this prevents discrimination.
- Clinical trials should be made as practical as possible for older people.
- Clinical trials should be safe for older people.
- Outcome measures should be relevant for older people.
- The values of older people participating in clinical trials should be respected.

be as practicable and safe as possible for older people; outcome measures should be relevant for older people; and the values of older people participating in trials should be respected.

5 **Future directions**

Trials have begun to look at the important issue of care of the old and frail. A good example is stroke treatment, including care in nursing homes rather than just in the hospital setting (44). Stroke often impairs executive function and mobility, which in turn interferes with the ability to perform activities of daily living. Because stroke victims may benefit from occupational therapy, a study has been designed to test this using suitable outcome measures (45); other work shows that cognitive rehabilitation interventions are also important (46). These studies focused on very basic questions about the impact of therapies on outcome measures relevant to the frail and elderly. Questions remain, but there are signs of an increasing body of research work investigating these important and practical areas of care.

However, many areas of care are less specific to the elderly, and it is here that problems persist. In spite of the fact that older people make up a substantial proportion of the population with a disease, they tend to be exluded from trials. For example, Cherubini et al. examined 251 trials investigating heart failure (16). Fully 25% excluded patients by placing an upper age limit, and 43% had at least one poorly justified exclusion. Analysis of Medicare beneficiaries for heart failure showed that 80% were over 65 years old, yet the SOLVD, MERIT-HF, and RALES studies recruited 18, 13, and 25%, respectively.

This persisting problem has been highlighted in Age UK's 'Understanding the Oldest Old' (2013) and by various EU attempts to develop good practice. Practical help with how to run clinical trials is provided by the document 'Medical Research for and with Older People in Europe'. Web links to these documents are given at end of the chapter.

The issue of under-representation particularly affects those with cognitive impairment (17,47) and even those with Parkinson's disease. This issue has been recognized by the NIHR (48), which has called for 'Equity in Clinical Research: Inclusion of Older Participants'. In the words of that document, 'Older people suffer the greatest burden of ill health in the Western world, yet are consistently under-represented in clinical trials'. Guidance on good practice in research has also been created with the aim of improving recruitment of older people (2).

It would seem self-evident that drugs should be tested on a population that represents the people who will receive the drug in clinical practice. One route to this is legislation. Depending on its wording, however, legislation can be a blunt tool with unpredictable outcomes.

The issue of under-representation is becoming recognized worldwide. Its impact goes beyond older people who receive the medication to the whole of society, because it is society that carries the burden of providing health and social care (49).

6 **Conclusion**

There has been some progress on the inclusion of older people in clinical trials, although more so in the USA than in Europe. Even so, there remains a fundamental lack of inclusion. We need the population taking part in clinical trials to match the age distribution of the diseases the therapies are designed to combat. The increasing proportion of older people in the population means that this is now a major priority.

Websites and guidelines relevant to this chapter

Medical research for and with older people in Europe proposed guidance for ethical aspects.

<http://www.efgcp.eu/%5Cdownloads%5CEFGCP%20Geriatric%20Research %20Guidelines%20Feb.2012%20for%20public%20consultation.pdf>

Age UK. Understanding the oldest old.

<http://www.ageuk.org.uk/Documents/EN-GB/For-professionals/Research/ Improving%20Later%20Life%202%20WEB.pdf?dtrk=true>

PREDICT (Increasing the participation of the elderly in clinical trials) website:

< http://www.predicteu.org>

PREDICT reports:

< http://www.predicteu.org/Reports/reports.html>

PREDICT charter:

<http://www.predicteu.org/PREDICT_Charter/predict_charter.html>

References

1 **Gu Q, Dillon CF, Burt VL.** Prescription drug use continues to increase: U.S. prescription drug data for 2007–2008. NCHS Data Brief. Sep;(42):1–8. National Center for Health Statistics. 2010. http://www.cdc.gov/nchs/data/databriefs/db42.pdf

2 **McMurdo ME, Roberts H, Parker S, Wyatt N, May H, Goodman C, et al.** Improving recruitment of older people to research through good practice. Age Ageing. 2011 Nov;**40**(6):659–65. PubMed PMID: 21911335.

3 **PREDICT WORKPACKAGE 1 2010.** http://www.predicteu.org/Reports/PREDICT_ WP1_Report.pdf

4 **Editorial.** Neurology in the elderly: more trials urgently needed. Lancet Neurol. 2009;**8**:969.

5 Cooke CR, Erickson SE, Watkins TR, Matthay MA, Hudson LD, Rubenfeld GD. Age-, sex-, and race-based differences among patients enrolled versus not enrolled in acute lung injury clinical trials. Crit Care Med. 2010 Jun;**38**(6):1450–7. PubMed PMID: 20386308.

6 Lee PY, Alexander KP, Hammill BG, Pasquali SK, Peterson ED. Representation of elderly persons and women in published randomized trials of acute coronary syndromes. JAMA-J Am Med Assoc. 2001 Aug 8;**286**(6):708–13. PubMed PMID: 11495621.

7 McMechan SR, Adgey AA. Age related outcome in acute myocardial infarction. Elderly people benefit from thrombolysis and should be included in trials. BMJ. 1998 Nov 14;**317**(7169):1334–5. PubMed PMID: 9812927. PubMed Central PMCID: 1114245.

8 Kitzman DW, Rich MW. Age disparities in heart failure research. JAMA-J Am Med Assoc. 2010 Nov 3;**304**(17):1950–1. PubMed PMID: 21045104. PubMed Central PMCID: 3685493.

9 Gurwitz JH, Magid DJ, Smith DH, Goldberg RJ, McManus DD, Allen LA, et al. Contemporary prevalence and correlates of incident heart failure with preserved ejection fraction. Am J Med. 2013 May;**126**(5):393–400. PubMed PMID: 23499328. PubMed Central PMCID: 3627730.

10 Cowie MR, Wood DA, Coats AJ, Thompson SG, Poole-Wilson PA, Suresh V, et al. Incidence and aetiology of heart failure; a population-based study. Europ Heart J. 1999 Mar;**20**(6):421–8. PubMed PMID: 10213345.

11 Masoudi FA, Havranek EP, Krumholz HM. The burden of chronic congestive heart failure in older persons: magnitude and implications for policy and research. Heart Failure Rev. 2002 Jan;**7**(1):9–16. PubMed PMID: 11790919.

12 Heiat A, Gross CP, Krumholz HM. Representation of the elderly, women, and minorities in heart failure clinical trials. Arch Internal Med. 2002 Aug 12–26;**162**(15): 1682–8. PubMed PMID: 12153370.

13 Bartlett C, Doyal L, Ebrahim S, Davey P, Bachmann M, Egger M, et al. The causes and effects of socio-demographic exclusions from clinical trials. Health Technol Assess. 2005 Oct;**9**(38):iii–iv, ix–x, 1–152. PubMed PMID: 16181564.

14 Crome P, Lally F, Cherubini A, Oristrell J, Beswick AD, Clarfield AM, et al. Exclusion of older people from clinical trials: professional views from nine European countries participating in the PREDICT study. Drugs Aging. 2011 Aug 1;**28**(8):667–77. PubMed PMID: 21812501.

15 Watts G. Why the exclusion of older people from clinical research must stop. BMJ. 2012;**344**:e3445. PubMed PMID: 22613873.

16 Cherubini A, Oristrell J, Pla X, Ruggiero C, Ferretti R, Diestre G, et al. The persistent exclusion of older patients from ongoing clinical trials regarding heart failure. Arch Internal Med. 2011 Mar 28;**171**(6):550–6. PubMed PMID: 21444844.

17 Fitzsimmons PR, Blayney S, Mina-Corkill S, Scott GO. Older participants are frequently excluded from Parkinson's disease research. Parkinsonism Rel Disorder. 2012 Jun;**18**(5):585–9. PubMed PMID: 22494661.

18 Bayer A, Tadd W. Unjustified exclusion of elderly people from studies submitted to research ethics committee for approval: descriptive study. BMJ. 2000 Oct 21;**321**(7267): 992–3. PubMed PMID: 11039965. PubMed Central PMCID: 27507.

19 Bugeja G, Kumar A, Banerjee AK. Exclusion of elderly people from clinical research: a descriptive study of published reports. BMJ. 1997 Oct 25;**315**(7115):1059. PubMed PMID: 9366735. PubMed Central PMCID: 2127695.

20 Cruz-Jentoft AJ, Gutiérrez B. Upper age limits in studies submitted to a research ethics committee. Aging Clin Exp Res. 2010;**22**:175–8.

21 Dixon-Woods M, Angell EL. Research involving adults who lack capacity: how have research ethics committees interpreted the requirements? J Med Ethics. 2009 Jun;**35**(6): 377–81. PubMed PMID: 19482983.

22 Department of Health. Guidance on nominating a consultee for research involving adults who lack capacity to consent. 22 Feb 2008. Issued by the Secretary of State and the Welsh Ministers in accordance with section 32(3) of the Mental Capacity Act 2005. http://webarchive.nationalarchives.gov.uk/20130107105354/http:/www.dh.gov.uk/en/Publicationsandstatistics/Publications/PublicationsPolicyAndGuidance/DH_083131

23 Townsley CA, Selby R, Siu LL. Systematic review of barriers to the recruitment of older patients with cancer onto clinical trials. J Clin Oncol. 2005 May 1;**23**(13):3112–24. PubMed PMID: 15860871.

24 Ross S, Grant A, Counsell C, Gillespie W, Russell I, Prescott R. Barriers to participation in randomised controlled trials: a systematic review. J Clin Epidemiol. 1999;**52**(12): 1143–56.

25 Beswick AD, Rees K, Griebsch I, Taylor FC, Burke M, West RR, Victory J, Brown J, Taylor RS, Ebrahim S. Provision, uptake and cost of cardiac rehabilitation programmes: improving services to under-represented groups. Health Technol Assess. 2004 Oct;**8**(41):iii–iv,ix–x,1–152.

26 Klabunde CN, Springer BC, Butler B, White MS, Atkins J. Factors influencing enrollment in clinical trials for cancer treatment. Southern Med J. 1999;**92**(12):1189–93.

27 Rendell JM, Merritt RK, Geddes JR. Incentives and disincentives to participation by clinicians in randomised controlled trials. Cochrane Methodology Review Group. Epub 2005 Jul 20. doi: 10.1002/14651858.MR000021

28 Townsley CA, Chan KK, Pond GR, Marquez C, Siu LL, Straus SE. Understanding the attitudes of the elderly towards enrolment into cancer clinical trials. BMC Cancer. 2006;**6**:34. PubMed PMID: 16466574. PubMed Central PMCID: 1382233.

29 Corbie-Smith G, Viscoli CM, Kernan WN, Brass LM, Sarrel P, Horwitz RI. Influence of race, clinical, and other socio-demographic features on trial participation. J Clin Epidemiol. 2003 Apr;**56**(4):304–9. PubMed PMID: 12767406.

30 Gross CP, Wong N, Dubin JA, Mayne ST, Krumholz HM. Enrollment of older persons in cancer trials after the Medicare reimbursement policy change. Arch Internal Med. 2005 Jul 11;**165**(13):1514–20. PubMed PMID: 16009867.

31 Sen Biswas M, Newby LK, Bastian LA, Peterson ED, Sugarman J. Who refuses enrollment in cardiac clinical trials? Clin Trials. 2007;**4**(3):258–63. PubMed PMID: 17715252.

32 Boles M, Getchell WS, Feldman G, McBride R, Hart RG. Primary prevention studies and the healthy elderly: evaluating barriers to recruitment. J Commun Health. 2000 Aug;**25**(4):279–92. PubMed PMID: 10941692.

33 Meropol NJ, Buzaglo JS, Millard J, Damjanov N, Miller SM, Ridgway C, et al. Barriers to clinical trial participation as perceived by oncologists and patients. J National Comprehensive Cancer Network: JNCCN. 2007 Sep;**5**(8):655–64. PubMed PMID: 17927923.

34 Kenyon S, Dixon-Woods M, Jackson CJ, Windridge K, Pitchforth E. Participating in a trial in a critical situation: a qualitative study in pregnancy. Qual Safety Health Care. 2006 Apr;**15**(2):98–101. PubMed PMID: 16585108. PubMed Central PMCID: 2464828.

35 **Le Quintrec JL, Piette F, Herve C.** [Clinical trials in very elderly people: the point of view of geriatricians]. Therapie. 2005 Mar-Apr;**60**(2):109–15. PubMed PMID: 15969313. Les essais therapeutiques chez les sujets tres ages: le point de vue des geriatres.

36 **Witham MD, McMurdo ME.** How to get older people included in clinical studies. Drugs Aging. 2007;**24**(3):187–96. PubMed PMID: 17362048.

37 **Baquet CR, Commiskey P, Daniel Mullins C, Mishra SI.** Recruitment and participation in clinical trials: socio-demographic, rural/urban, and health care access predictors. Cancer Detect Prevent. 2006;**30**(1):24–33. PubMed PMID: 16495020. PubMed Central PMCID: 3276312.

38 **Watson JM, Torgerson DJ.** Increasing recruitment to randomised trials: a review of randomised controlled trials. BMC Med Res Methodol. 2006;**6**:34. PubMed PMID: 16854229. PubMed Central PMCID: 1559709.

39 **Donovan J, Mills N, Smith M, Brindle L, Peters T, et al.** Quality improvement report: improving design and conduct of randomised trials by embedding them in qualitative research: ProtecT (prostate testing for cancer and treatment) study. BMJ. 2002;**325**(7367):766–70.

40 **Harris TJ, Carey IM, Victor CR, Adams R, Cook DG.** Optimising recruitment into a study of physical activity in older people: a randomised controlled trial of different approaches. Age Ageing. 2008 Nov;**37**(6):659–65. PubMed PMID: 18718924.

41 **Rahman M, Morita S, Fukui T, Sakamoto J.** Physicians' reasons for not entering their patients in a randomized controlled trial in Japan. Tohoku J Experiment Med. 2004 Jun;**203**(2):105–9. PubMed PMID: 15212145.

42 **Sellors J, Cosby R, Trim K, Kaczorowski J, Howard M, Hardcastle L, et al.** Recruiting family physicians and patients for a clinical trial: lessons learned. Family Practice. 2002 Feb;**19**(1):99–104. PubMed PMID: 11818358.

43 **The PREDICT EU Charter: European Charter for Older People in Clinical Trials 2011.** http://www.predicteu.org/PREDICT_Charter/predict_charter.html

44 **Fletcher-Smith JC, Walker MF, Cobley CS, Steultjens EM, Sackley CM.** Occupational therapy for care home residents with stroke. Cochrane Database Syst Rev. 2013;6:CD010116. PubMed PMID: 23740541.

45 **Sackley CM, Burton CR, Herron-Marx S, Lett K, Mant J, Roalfe AK, et al.** A cluster randomised controlled trial of an occupational therapy intervention for residents with stroke living in UK care homes (OTCH): study protocol. BMC Neurol. 2012;**12**:52. PubMed PMID: 22776066. PubMed Central PMCID: 3436864.

46 **Chung CS, Pollock A, Campbell T, Durward BR, Hagen S.** Cognitive rehabilitation for executive dysfunction in adults with stroke or other adult non-progressive acquired brain damage. Cochrane Database Syst Rev. 2013;4:CD008391. PubMed PMID: 23633354.

47 **Taylor JS, DeMers SM, Vig EK, Borson S.** The disappearing subject: exclusion of people with cognitive impairment and dementia from geriatrics research. J Am Geriatr Soc. 2012 Mar;**60**(3):413–9. PubMed PMID: 22288835.

48 **National Institute for Health Research Clinical Research Coordinating Centre Age and Ageing Specialty Group.** Equity in clinical research: inclusion of older participants. 2010. www.crncc.nihr.ac.uk/Resources/NIHR%20CRN%20CC/Documents/equity_in_clinical_research_22June2010.pdf

49 **McMurdo M.** Clinical research must include more older people. BMJ. 2013;**346**(f3899).

Index